ALZHEIMERS

What it is,
how to cope

ISOBELLE GIDLEY
& RICHARD SHEARS

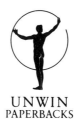

UNWIN
PAPERBACKS

LONDON SYDNEY WELLINGTON

First published in paperback by Unwin ® Paperbacks,
an imprint of Unwin Hyman Limited, in 1988
Reprinted 1989

First published in Australia
by Unwin Paperbacks 1987

UNWIN HYMAN LTD
15/17 Broadwick Street
London W1V 1FP

UNWIN ® PAPERBACKS
Allen & Unwin Australia Pty Ltd
8 Napier Street, North Sydney, NSW 2060, Australia

Unwin Paperbacks New Zealand Pty Ltd with
Port Nicholson Press
75 Ghuznee Street, Wellington, New Zealand

ISBN 0 04 614005 0.

Typeset in Garamond by Asco Trade Typesetting
Limited, Hong Kong

Produced by SRM Production Services Sdn Bhd, Malaysia

CONTENTS

FOREWORD

In the autumn of 1979 I found out my mother was suffering from irreversible dementia or, more specifically, Alzheimer's disease. Finally, after seven years of toil and despair, of hope and frustration, of helplessly watching her sink deeper and deeper into a chasm of forgetfulness and physical decay, a name had been given to the monster that consumed her.

We had taken her to a number of specialists who duly prescribed enormous doses of medication, their conclusions, without exception, having been 'hardening of the arteries or high blood-pressure' and even 'nothing wrong'. But something was definitely amiss. So, finding the medical profession unable to help we turned to witch-doctors, spiritual healers, Filipino psychic surgeons, Indian holy men, magicians, homeopaths and polarising therapists, massaging, dieting and fasting her. To no avail ... she continued to decline.

Her lovely eyes were now two hard, disembodied, glittering stones. Sometimes she acted as if possessed by some evil force. Once the epitome of grace and manners, she greedily consumed everything and anything: paper, tinfoil, soap, plastic, flowers. She defecated and urinated in secret corners and behind neighbours' shrubs — she was so totally disoriented we didn't dare let her out of sight. 'Friends' melted away, whispering she was mad, that she ought to be committed; meeting our attempts to care for her at home, to treat her as normal, with scorn and derision. But we refused to give in and refused to let her give in, and instead filled her life with more colour, more music, more poetry and more love whenever criticism was strongest.

I would not accept that nothing could be done and set off on a fact-finding mission that took in the world. Later, Richard joined me. In a way, we are living out a fairytale. There is Madeline, bewitched, and the rest of us who love her must undergo innumerable trials in order to break the spell. The biggest test is to retain good cheer, honour and integrity and to be able to move with the alchemic changes which just might transform lead into gold. Madeline is joined with us in this dance of life. It matters not that she has forgotten the steps; it is up to us to lead her as the music changes from waltz to foxtrot and even to a disco beat ... but that personal odyssey is another story.

This book is for Madeline and all the others who have fallen prey to the same monster. It is also for those who care for them and the professionals who search out the answers. My one regret is we never said goodbye ...

Isobelle Gidley
Melbourne, 1985

PREFACE

At the outset, we were aware that researching and preparing a book on Alzheimer's disease and related brain disorders would be a formidable task. Almost daily, medical investigation takes a step forward in one laboratory, a stride back in another. How far into the past should we look? How far into the future? Should we be hopeful that one day what is known as irreversible dementia will be prevented? Or should we take the line suggested by several neurologists that prevention, and certainly cure, are so far away that a child born today has a chance of ending his years with a dead mind?

It would be misleading to dismiss the negative, for it would mean ignoring the painstaking work of those who have searched for and, for the moment, failed to find the answers; and it would be turning a deaf ear to the grief and frustration of families who live with a dementing relative. But we obviously could not overlook the hopes of many medical researchers. For a start, the strange brain formations described by Alois Alzheimer are now seen to be a disease and are under specific investigation, whereas a few years ago 'senility' and its associated loss of faculties was accepted as a normal process of ageing.

We decided to take no particular line, but present both promise and despair. Certainly, as medical research into the disease stands today, no cures or proven preventative measures can be suggested, and we face the possibility of heading into the twenty-first century with a significant proportion of the population suffering irreversible dementia. This is going to place great strain on the social, political and economic fabric of our society. Who will care for these people? As is the case in most western countries, the government will be expected to take on the responsibility of providing. But because proper care is labour-intensive and costly, will there be an increasing trend to find other means of dealing with the problem? Today, drugs are widely used with the tacit approval of the medical profession and the general population. Will attitudes change to permit voluntary and perhaps even involuntary euthanasia? Medical opinions vary, and we have struck many different viewpoints when researching this book. To avoid tedium, we decided to base our information on general assessment. Most of our research was carried out in the United States, Britain and Australia, but data have been gathered from other countries including Holland, Germany, Sweden and Canada. Information from other nations is still being collated and will possibly be published later; for the sake of expediency, we felt that the present manuscript should be released now.

This is not a textbook, so we do not make specific citations, although all sources are listed. And we ensure that throughout the book opinions and research findings are attributed to those who made them. As a point of presentation, we generally refer to afflicted individuals by the male gender, the grammatically standard form, although the majority of sufferers are women.

We found enthusiasm for the book wherever we travelled, and assistance came from all quarters — the medical profession, social workers, governments and families who have a dementia victim in their midst. Most family members asked for anonymity, and their wishes are respected. To all who encouraged us — librarians, secretaries, doctors, nurses, friends and many more — we express our deep gratitude.

Particular thanks are accorded to Jim Novy and Mary Sweeny, Alzheimer's Disease and Related Disorders Association Inc., 360 North Michigan Avenue, Chicago, Illinois; US Department of Health and Human Services, especially the Office of Scientific and Health Reports; National Institute of Neurological and Communicative Disorders and Stroke at the National Institutes of Health, Bethesda, Maryland; Alzheimer's Disease Centre, Albert Einstein College of Medicine, 1300 Morris Park Avenue, Bronx, New York 10461; The Burke Rehabilitation Centre, 785 Mamaroneck Avenue, White Plains, New York 10605; Community Health Information Network, Community Health Education Department, Mt Auburn Hospital, Cambridge, Massachusetts 02138; Department of Psychiatry and Behavioral Sciences, University of Washington, Seattle; Department of Neuropathology, Radcliffe Infirmary, Oxford, England.

Christine Davis, projects officer, and library staff at the Kings Fund Centre, 126 Albert Street, London NW1 7NF; Terri Spy and

Isobel Ludley of the Alzheimer's Disease Society, Bank Buildings, Fulham Broadway, London SW6; Brian Moss, Director, Moorfields Community for Adult Care, 20–26 Manningtree Road, Hawthorn, Victoria 3122, Australia; Henry Brodaty, Jane Byrne and Roy Hambley of the Alzheimer's Disease and Related Disorders Society, PO Box K365, Haymarket, Sydney, NSW 2000; Miriam Hirschfield, Department of Nursing, Sackler School of Medicine, School of Continuing Medical Education, Tel Aviv University, Israel; Community Care Centre, Royal Southern Memorial Hospital, Caulfield, Melbourne; Bethia Hays, Melbourne; Alzheimer's Disease and Related Disorders Society of Victoria, c/o Victorian Association for Mental Health, 107 Rathdowne Street, Carlton, Victoria 3053; Department of Health, NSW; Dr Cees van Tiggelen, Victoria, Australia; Barbara Janes, Montefiore Hospital and Medical Centre, 111 East 210th Street, Bronx, New York; Patricia Jacobs, US Department of Agriculture Human Nutrition Research Center on Ageing at Tufts University, Boston, Mass.; Ruth Mushin, Community Development Officer, Ethnic Communities' Council of Victoria.

We have found background and other material written by Robert N. Butler, M.D., former director, and Marian Emr, public information specialist, at the National Institute on Ageing, Washington, DC, particularly helpful. We are also very grateful to Judy MacLean, editor of *Generations*, the Journal of the Western Gerontological Society, 833 Market Street, San Francisco, Calif. 94103, for permission to use material written by Miriam K. Aronson, Ed.D.; Robert Katzman, M.D.; Nancy Neveloff Dubler, LL.B.; Robert N. Butler, M.D.; Marian Emr; Steven S. Matsuyama, Ph.D. and Lissy F. Jarvik, M.D., Ph.D.; Ira Katz, M.D., Ph.D.; Rochelle Lipkowitz, R.N., M.S.; Peter H. Millard, M.D.; Barbara Silverstone, D.S.W.; Deborah Bookin; Carl Eisdorfer, M.D., Ph.D.; Donna Cohen, Ph.D.; Jerome H. Stone; Mrs Bobbie Glaze; and Warren Easterly.

Thanks are also accorded to our editor, Matthew Kelly, for his enthusiasm and support while we were researching and writing this book.

We accept there are areas we have not touched and family problems we have not uncovered, but we feel that if this book goes some way towards enlightening the public about dementia, some good will have come from it.

1

The human brain

The human brain, storehouse of memory, emotion and reason, is the most complex portion of the nervous system. Yet it is so wonderful, so complicated, that many of its secrets remain locked away from the most probing of microscopes. Little wonder that early man regarded it as a magic box. The ancient Greeks and Romans, awestruck by its reservoir of information, compared its functions to those of their baths, fountains and aqueducts. Lenin's mind fascinated Russian scientists so much that after his death his brain was removed, then dissected and studied for more than two years while neurologists searched for some clue to his intellect. At the World's Fair in New York in the mid-1960s, 61 kilometres of electrical wiring, whirring motors, tens of thousands of electric bulbs and twisting tubes were carefully linked to depict a giant electrified model of the human brain, yet the scientific advisers pointed out that 'it's nothing like as complicated as the real thing'.

The pinkish-grey brain, floating in protective shock-absorbing fluid, is the most astounding creation on earth. It never rests, even when we are sleeping or day dreaming, continually consuming oxygen and glucose from the blood. It requires about a fifth of the blood that is pumped through the heart, and it consumes some 20 per cent of the oxygen used by the body. Close to 800 mL of blood flows through the brain every minute, and 75 mL is always present. Early scientists who tried to fathom the intricate workings were denounced for treading on forbidden territory, being accused of heresy. But in time, with the announcement of important discoveries, the medical investigators were acknowledged and lauded.

We now know that the fully developed brain contains something like 12 billion nerve cells — neurons — which are packed in with, and greatly outnumbered by, other cells called glias. These work in harmony with billions of nerve cell fibres running through the body and act in such a way as to give us our character and individuality. Our eyes see pictures; our ears pick up sounds. These messages are absorbed by the brain, being passed from neuron to neuron. The nerve cells act like electrical points, providing their own power to pass the message on, but the transmission is through a chemical, not by electricity. When a signal is being sent, it crosses a junction known as a synapse, leaving a fibre called an axon on the transmitting cell and being received by a branch-like arm — a dendrite — projecting from the receiving cell. If we could imagine a single neuron enlarged to the size of a cricket ball, the axon would be more than a mile long (about 2 kilometres) and the branches of the receiving dendrite would fill London's Albert Hall or the Sydney Opera House.

The message is channelled to areas that enable us to identify language, music or everyday sounds. Other parts convert that which our eyes see into pictures or make us yell when we feel pain or smile when we hear good news. Whenever we are conscious, looking, hearing, feeling, our axons and dendrites are bristling with activity. Minute after minute, week after week, year after year, information is relayed through that amazing cell structure and, depending on the character of the individual brain, the pictures or words will be stored for instant recall or be pushed into some dark passage to fade for all time. The minute information the brain is capable of retaining for decades is astonishing. A lifetime on, we might recall the name of our maths teacher, see his face, remember the colour of his jacket. Some extraordinary feats of memory have been reported in scientific journals, among them the case of a builder who, under hypnosis, was able to recall every mark, every bump, on a brick he put in a wall some twenty years earlier.

Despite the difference in sizes of brains — in the 1800s scientists measured and weighed the brains of famous men to seek a common denominator — weight has nothing to do with intelligence. The brain of a genius will still be about 1000–1500 gm, or some 2 per cent of the total body weight, no heavier or lighter than that of the proverbial village idiot. But why some brains are sharper than others is unknown.

When working properly, the brain is a remarkable control box, responsible for the movement of every muscle, every blink of an eye, every tear. But if anything impedes its operation, we see the effects in the body; disorders of the brain bring on the most profound human misery. A stroke, which occurs when a blood vessel is blocked and an area of brain dies (producing an infarct), can result in the transmission system being impaired. A less common stroke results when a blood vessel bursts, causing bleeding into the brain. The effect in either case is interference with motor functions — movements of arms and legs — and the victim is paralysed, perhaps down one side of the body. A blow on the head can also cause a blood clot, which puts pressure on the brain and affects functions such as speech and fast reflexes. Damage this precious, priceless commodity and the harmed part will remain dead, for neurons do not replace themselves.

As we age, our brains shrink and lose weight and we approach the end of our lives with many less cells than in our youth. This can affect our memories to some extent, and speech might be slower. But generally our brains, if unaffected by accident, misadventure or disease will 'see us out'.

For an unfortunate number of people, the reverse will happen. Their brains will break down while their bodies remain healthy. They will slowly change from 'normal' people into bewildered, confused, helpless beings. For inexplicable reasons, something will happen to their brains. A creeping malady of no known origin will sabotage those vital cells, turning the source of life and thought into a useless lump of matter. A global tragedy, it leads us towards the new century.

2

Identifying
Alzheimer's disease

*Ross MacDonald, whose tightly written
novels about the hard-boiled private eye
Lew Archer lifted the modern detective
novel to the level of literature, died of
Alzheimer's disease Monday night in Santa
Barbara, Calif. He was 67 years old... For
more than three years he had been suffering
from Alzheimer's disease, which causes devastating changes in the brain and progressive mental deterioration.*
— *New York Times*, Wednesday
13 July 1983

With this newspaper account, Alzheimer's disease touched the
masses for the first time. A personality had died not from a stroke
or a heart attack or cancer but from the effects of a withered mind.

That the prestigious *New York Times* had officially recorded
Alzheimer's disease as the cause of MacDonald's death was, indeed,
a sign of the times. His obituary was carried on a page shared by
men who had died for more generally known reasons — an ex-
mayor who had suffered a heart attack, a former congressman who
had succumbed to his road crash injuries, a cancer researcher who
tragically had become a victim of lung cancer. On that same
Wednesday, hundreds of others, not well known enough to warrant obituaries in the national papers around the world, died of
strokes and cancers and injuries and, although the name might not
have been written on their death certificates, of Alzheimer's disease. Often the cause of death in Alzheimer cases is officially
described as pneumonia, and although that might be the ultimate

reason for life ending, the root of the problem has been a brain so twisted and tangled that it has been unable to control the body's immune system.

It is an unfortunate fact of life that it has taken the affliction of the famous to draw attention to a disease that can strike anyone from the age of 40 onwards, and in some cases even younger. Film star Rita Hayworth, pin-up queen of the Second World War, has been ravaged by the disease, and it has taken her illness to enlighten another former film star, Ronald Reagan, President of the United States, about its worldwide destruction of the human mind. In a letter from the White House to Miss Hayworth's daughter, Princess Yasmin Aga Khan, he wrote:

'Like most Americans, my true understanding of the tragedy called Alzheimer's disease is relatively recent. For too long this insidious, indiscriminate killer of mind and life has gone undetected, while the families of its victims have gone unaided ...'

President Reagan was not unfamiliar with the disease when he wrote that. For his own mother was an Alzheimer sufferer, eventually succumbing to a stroke at the age of 80. Although there are strong indications that the affliction can be passed down through families, the President's physician, Dr Daniel Ruge, says: 'You can take it from me — the President doesn't have it.' Nevertheless, when he was sworn in, Reagan pledged to step down if he detected any signs of senility in himself. Interestingly, prior to his reelection in November 1984, Reagan's public speeches caught the attention of a British speech analyst who considered the President's speech patterns indicated the early stages of senility. Dr Brian Butterworth of London's University College listened carefully to Reagan's second debate with Walter Mondale, then declared: 'It seems that President Reagan is much less competent at speaking than he was four years ago when he was debating Carter. These indications of decline seem to be consistent with a diagnosis of early stages of senility.' In the President's first debate with Mondale, he made 'badly constructed sentences, sentences which aren't grammatical, sentences which are cut off in the middle'. When Reagan debated Carter in 1980 he made one of these errors every 1000 words, which is within the normal range. Now it was close to one in every 200 words.

The disease has crept into film scripts to add real human tragedy to the plot. An episode of the television series 'Trapper John, M.D.'

entitled 'Forget Me Not' showed a young surgeon with the early symptoms of Alzheimer's disease. He knew what his fate would be, and after a period of denial he accepted it. Another TV series, 'Hill Street Blues' has Mick 'Dog Breath' Belker telling his friend that his father has Alzheimer's disease, and later it is revealed Mick's father dies of 'pneumonia', often the ultimate cause of death for an afflicted person. In Holland in 1984, when a doctor gave a talk on television about the disease, more than 20 000 viewers swamped the switchboard begging for more information.

Alzheimer's disease is now officially recognised as the fourth biggest natural killer after heart attacks, cancers and strokes. The United States Department of Health and Human Services, in a special scientific guide for health practitioners, acknowledges that in America alone Alzheimer's disease is responsible for an estimated 100 000 to 120 000 deaths a year. Yet as recently as 1977, although there were more than two million deaths in the United States, only 2117 were recorded as being caused by Alzheimer's disease.

In Britain, one person in ten over the age of 65 is mentally impaired by what is known as senile dementia, a class of mental conditions in which Alzheimer's disease is included. Professor A.N. Exton-Smith, a dementia expert at London's University College, says that during the next fifteen years the number of people over 85 is likely to increase by 45 per cent. This is the group most likely to succumb to dementia. 'The sheer magnitude of the problem will be a great challenge to medical practice,' he says. And the British Health Advisory Service, in a 1983 report outlining the burgeoning problem of a growing elderly population, says: 'Unless the challenges are met, the flood is likely to overwhelm the entire health care system ...'

A year earlier, the Secretary of State for Health and Social Services, Mr Norman Fowler, had presented Britain with a frightening picture. Since the mid-1960s, the numbers of those aged 65 had increased vastly, so that there were now seven million people in this age group — 1 800 000 more than in 1961. 'Over the next twenty years', he warned, 'we shall see equally dramatic changes, not so much in the overall numbers, but in the proportion of the particularly old.'

During this period, the number of people aged between 65 and 74 in Britain will actually decline by about half a million. But the daunting prediction is that those *over* the age of 75 will increase to more than three million, and those aged 85 and more will rise by 50 per cent to nearly three-quarters of a million by the end of the century. With an increase in its aged population Britain, too, faces the prospect of thousands more falling victim to Alzheimer's disease.

The problems are not so much an increasing aged population. We would all like to think that we can live longer, healthier lives. The frightening equation is that the longer we live, the greater our chances of falling victim to this incurable ailment.

Britain and America are not alone. Throughout Europe, as more people develop the disease, welfare workers shake their heads at the future picture: the elderly population will swell, and so will the number of problems. In West Germany, where the disease was first identified and defined, doctors throw up their hands and admit: 'We have no answers. It is still beating us.' The country is experiencing a big rise in the proportion of its elderly — about 13 per cent — and health workers concede that great difficulties lie ahead. Elderly people with mental problems in West Germany are cared for by the Mental Health Authority, but officials admit that while a real problem exists, a solution is uncertain.

On the other side of the world, in Australia, where incredible advances have been made in 'test tube baby' research, the figure has been put as high as one elderly person in six suffering from dementia, a total of some 100 000. Such figures prompted Dr P.M. Last, a medical coordinator in the South Australian Health Commission, to tell a national hospital congress that mental deterioration presented a 'major challenge' to governments.

Medical scientists have been able to take great strides in helping to bring healthy babies into the world, but they can offer little for adults whose last years on earth are confused, frightening and, in many cases, undignified. Will those 'miracle babies', whose births would have been impossible a few years earlier, finish their lives 50, 60, 70 years on, fragmented and more helpless than the day they were born? It is not an impossible prospect, for to cure Alzheimer's disease is, at the moment, a task beyond the skills of all medical scientists, many accepting that a cure may never be found.

The implications for future governments are enormous. Dr Robert Butler, former director of the US National Institute on Ageing and now in charge of the department of geriatrics at the Mount Sinai School of Medicine, estimates that by 1990 about

US $30 billion — nearly half the nation's estimated total nursing home bill — will be spent to institutionalise people with Alzheimer's disease or other forms of dementia.

'The triumph of this century in making it possible for people to live longer makes even more poignant the fact that one of the fallouts of long life for some people is the vulnerability to this devastating disease,' he says. 'I want to say that in a qualified manner, because clearly if 4 or 6 per cent develop the disease, then something like 95 per cent don't have it. But in absolute numbers, or as a proportion, it's just astronomical, especially since numbers of older persons in this country alone are growing daily by 1600 persons and roughly 600 000 a year.

'So that if we don't find some remedies, some forms of prevention, some effective ways of treatment of senile dementia of the Alzheimer's type, we're going to have an incredible burgeoning of the nursing home population, enormous anguish in families, great and escalating costs and, I fear, the prospect of some coldbloodedness.'

'Sometimes', says a 40-year-old professional man working in Melbourne, 'I wonder how my wife holds off from killing her mother. Her mother has nothing left. All day she sits dribbling and peeing in her pants. The only thing she does to help is open her mouth to be fed. My wife is so courageous and everybody says how wonderful she is to be doing this job, but nobody really knows what it's like when they all go away and the door closes. They don't know that after being a slave to a living corpse throughout the day, my wife has to change the sheets on her mother's bed two and three times a night sometimes; nobody else hears the old lady's screams and groans throughout the night. Nobody really sees the love mixed with pain in my wife's eyes. Nobody has seen her drop to the floor and cry, cry, cry, her back breaking, her arms aching from lugging her mother to the lavatory, back to her chair, to the lavatory, back to the chair, hour after hour, day after day, week after week. Nobody has seen her on her hands and knees in the bathroom scrubbing up faeces which have got everywhere because of her mother's incontinence. People who come to visit only see a spotless, odour-free house with an elderly lady sitting in a chair. It's because my wife is burning away her own young life to keep the place like that, keep her mother clean and dignified, that nobody really knows how bad it is. When I see my wife with her head in her arms and I hear her sobs, I think, how easy it would be to finish the agony for her. How easy it would be to leave her mother in a draught so she gets pneumonia. Would it be murder or the ultimate kindness — kindness for the two of them? I know I wouldn't have the guts to do it, and what right do I have, because she is not my mother. But I wonder sometimes why my wife isn't moved to it. I tell you, when somebody's brain gets eaten away like her mother's it's a terrible, terrible thing.'

In 1981 a report by the British Royal College of Physicians acknowledged that institutional care was unlikely to expand and most demented elderly would have to be cared for in their own homes. This would cast burdens on families and neighbourhoods as well as voluntary and hospital services. But, said the report, if home care was to be successful, near-universal re-education would be required. Even in 1981, the cost of keeping a person in an institution was enormous: £7500 a year.

As Dr Butler says, more families will cry out for help from the state. Our politicians will fall into an older age bracket, with the result that a higher percentage of them will be at risk from Alzheimer's disease. Unless a cure is found, a large proportion of the world's population will become the undead; alive in body, dead in mind. Of all human diseases, it is the most insidious, for it strips away all dignity, all finesse. It erodes beauty, turns geniuses into incomprehensible child-people and pulls families down to their knees, filling their lives with tears and despair and taking them to the edge of financial ruin.

Mr Lewis Thomas, Chancellor of New York's Memorial Sloane-Kettering Cancer Center, describes dementia as a disease of the century: 'the worst of all disease, not just for what it does to the victim but for its devastating effects on family and friends... It is, unmercifully, not lethal; patients go on and on living, essentially brainless but otherwise healthy, into advanced age, unless lucky enough to be saved by pneumonia.'

A disease of the century it may well be, yet paradoxically it casts us back to the Dark Ages with families being ashamed to admit they have someone in their midst with a disturbed mind.

An American brain expert, Dr Michael Shelanski of the Harvard Medical School, believes that failure to view ageing of the brain as a pathological process, a disease, will turn 'victories in our crusades against cancer and heart disease into hollow shells, and the fruits

of those victories will be bitter ones as we watch the wards of
our hospitals fill with older people who have strong bodies but
diminished minds.'

With such awesome problems ahead, the subject of euthanasia —
literally meaning a good, or painless, death — has sparked furious
debate. Should hopelessly demented people be allowed to live on,
casting an enormous burden on relatives and the community and
giving nothing but heartache in return? Relatives who have loved
that person for a lifetime and who still remember the best times are
appalled at any suggestion of an 'early' death. How, say others, can
euthanasia be brought about in dementia cases? It isn't possible to
'pull out the plug' or cease medication as in other terminal illness
cases and allow the person to die naturally. For a dementing person
to die earlier than his or her life expectancy would mean a deliberate act of terminating life, which becomes murder. Cutting down
on intensive personal care at home, either through the inability to
provide the services required or by deliberate neglect, might be regarded as a form of 'slow' euthanasia, as might committing a person
to a third-rate institution. Many people believe a 'compromise' is
the answer. They say drugs should be administered where necessary to help the inflicted retain dignity — tranquillisers, for example, to prevent shouting — but the course of nature ought to be
allowed to continue when those drugs do nothing more than prolong problems for both sufferer and carer.

In some quarters, opinions sound cruelly inhuman. In 1984, the
Governor of Colorado, Richard D. Lamm, caused a national out-
cry, his words rocking the Western world, when he remarked that
elderly people who are teminally ill have a 'duty to die and get out
of the way' instead of trying to prolong their lives by artificial
means. Senior citizen groups were furious, but Lamm was not hit-
ting against all the aged, only those whose lives are hopelessly sliding away, yet who continue to hang on with the help of machines,
devoted relatives and vast financial imput.

America's former Health, Education and Welfare Secretary,
Joseph A. Califano, Jr., is also concerned about the drain imposed
on medical resources by those who have gone beyond the point of
helping themselves. 'What do you do with someone who is senile
or has Alzheimer's disease, or for one reason or other cannot live
without another person helping him?' he asks. 'Let me give you a
sense of how urgent I think the problem is, and how politically

explosive I think it's going to become. I'm talking about what it means when you combine the long-term health-care problem — what do you do with somebody who is 85 years old and essentially not functioning but physically alive? — with the problem of the extraordinary cost of life-extending equipment.'

Califano points out that one-third of America's Medicare is spent on people with less than a year of life left to them, a cost of some $25 billion. He now believes that euthanasia will become the next searing issue, like abortion is today. 'It's going to be a burning, burning issue.'

He adds: 'We take care of a phenomenal proportion of our people. But we're going to have to take care of them in different ways in the future.

'The problems are that, one, our health care is too expensive, and, two, there are incredible changes taking place in our population in terms of the larger proportion of our people who are senior citizens. They consume most of the health care. Within that group particularly, there is a much larger number of people who are living to be much older.'

The life expectancy in the United States, he says, is about 72 for a man and 77 or 78 for a woman. However, those living to 65 have an expectancy of 81 or 82. Those later years tend to be more expensive because of the cost of doctors and machines and long-term care.

The victims of irreversible dementia step beyond the realms of sanity and never look back. There is only one road and it is a steady downhill slope. Families mourn the passing of the person they once knew, but the sorrow never ends because the husband, wife, parent, lives on. 'Caring for an Alzheimer's victim,' says one wife, 'is like a funeral that never ends.' There will be many more continuous funerals before the crying stops, for the unmerciful affliction continues to strike at random. Just what on God's earth is it?

Alzheimer's disease gets its name from a burly monocled German physician who told the world about the disease in 1906. One of Alois Alzheimer's patients in Tubingen was a middle-aged woman who, since 1902, had shown what he described as 'progressive jealousy' while at the same time she gradually lost her memory. Intellectually, she went downhill, became disorientated and hallucinated until finally she was unable to care for her bodily needs. When the woman died, Alzheimer decided to have a detailed look at her brain. She was just 51 years old, yet she had suffered symptoms associated with people in their eighties and nineties — people who were, in fact, victims of senile dementia. Senile dementia literally means old and deprived of mind. The inability to reason had been seen many times in elderly patients, and doctors had accepted this as something that happened to an unfortunate percentage in the last years and months of their lives. But how, Alzheimer asked, could anyone be senile in middle age?

Working in his laboratory with the aid of a couple of assistants, the neurologist opened the woman's skull and was surprised at the appearance of her brain. For a start, it was severely withered, looking as if it had dried up and shrunk. Everyone loses brain cells during their lifetime, but this patient's loss had been so great that the physical appearance of the brain had changed. The inner spaces of the woman's brain — the ventricles — were larger than normal, while the outer layer of cells was thinner than it should have been.

Surprised to find such 'wear' in the brain of a relatively young woman, Alzheimer made a more detailed study under the microscope. He saw that the nerve cells in the outer layer of the brain — the cerebral cortex — were riddled with jumbled-up fibres at the nerve endings, resembling tangled strands of wool. Alzheimer gave these jumbled fibres a name — neurofibrillary tangles, literally meaning nerve fibre tangles.

The physician noticed a second abnormality, which can clearly be seen by modern doctors using sophisticated instruments such as the electron microscope, which can magnify cells more than a hundred thousand times. With the aid of a tissue stain, Alzheimer saw that on the outside of the nerve cells there were deteriorating pieces of nerve cells grouped around a fibrous core. These are now known as neuritic plaques.

One brain pathologist describes the plaques as being similar to mothholes in cloth, and the tangles are as if someone has sliced through telephone cables with an axe. Another likens the interior of an Alzheimer brain to the aftermath of someone running amok in there with a shotgun. The plaques, it is known, interrupt the passage of signals in the brain, as if the brain is short-circuiting, cutting off memory messages and destroying the free flow of thought.

Alzheimer wasn't quite sure what the effects of the tangles were, and even now specialists can only guess that they constipate the nerve cells so that they gradually wind down. One noticeable effect on the brain is a decrease in a substance known as acetylcholine, which is essential for communication between nerve cells. The amount of this substance is reduced in a brain afflicted by Alzheimer's disease. Uncertain about the cause of the chemical changes, what Alzheimer did know was that in his laboratory he had the brain of a middle-aged woman and it could have been taken from a 90-year-old. Although he had made a remarkable discovery, he was not the first to recognise the disturbing behaviour of someone with a progressive brain disease.

Sixty-eight years earlier, in 1838, Dr Jean Esquirol, a prominent French physician, told his colleagues about *demence senile*, senile dementia. He described it as an illness that resulted in a loss of short-term memory, willpower and drive. It came on gradually and could be accompanied by emotional disturbances. Dr Esquirol's findings, however, were limited. For he described the condition as affecting only people over 65.

Yet Alzheimer identified a victim of exactly the same affliction and who was fourteen years younger than Esquirol's dividing line. In her case, it was not 'old age' dementia but 'pre-senile' dementia. However, the German was not aware that the condition he and Dr Esquirol had described a lifetime earlier were exactly the same thing.

Fifty years went by following Alzheimer's discoveries, with very little research undertaken on the disorder. At last, in the 1960s, three English scientists decided to take up where Alzheimer left off. Dr Bernard Tomlinson, Sir Martin Roth and Dr Garry Blessed selected 50 patients over the age of 65 who were obviously losing their minds. The idea was to wait until they died and then carry out post-mortem examinations on their brains. They also removed the brains of 28 people of the same ages who died in the same period but who were not demented. The scientists found that the brains of more than half the demented group had undergone the pathological changes identified by Alois Alzheimer — there were abnormal fibres and degenerated nerve endings. Compared with the brains of those who had not shown any outward symptoms of memory loss or lack of control, the differences were enormous. The scientists concluded that because the characteristics in the brains of the demented patients were exactly as described by Alzheimer after his examination of the 51-year-old, senile dementia and pre-senile dementia had to be the same thing. In other words, those whose brains became tangled before the age of 65 and those who developed the problem after that age all shared the disease which now carried Alzheimer's name.

The English scientists' findings fascinated their colleagues around the world. It had been a relatively simple survey, yet it was heralded as a great step forward. Research into the disease — for it was seen as a disease and not just a natural process of ageing — escalated. But apart from confirming time and again that when people develop tangles and plaques they lose control of their minds and bodies, researchers have not taken us much further along the discovery trail. They have, however, been able to establish that the tangles Alzheimer found are at their thickest around a part of the brain known as the hippocampus, where memories of recent events are believed to be stored. This area is also associated with the emotions. Doctors assume, then, that when their patient becomes progressively forgetful and show uncharacteristic emotions, something is happening up there in the hippocampus region. If the condition worsens, it is usually a sure sign that cell changes are occurring and that the fibres are becoming tangled. However, doctors cannot be certain about a diagnosis until after death when a post-mortem examination is carried out.

Yet the more research that is undertaken, the more confusing the situation becomes. Take those neuritic plaques, for example.... The US Health and Human Services Department acknowledges that when analysed, they have raised more questions about Alzheimer's disease than they have answered. At the centre of each plaque is a substance which has been called amyloid, an abnormal protein not usually present in the brain. This amyloid might be a clue to the root of the problem, or it could be a red herring. When amyloids form, scientists have learned, they are usually in the presence of a highly reactive type of molecule fragments which combine readily with other molecule pieces. Some scientists have formed the opinion that these 'gadabout' molecule fragments are the chief culprits in ageing because they bring about chemical reactions that lead to damage to vessels and cells right through the body. The amyloid core at the centre of each neuritic plaque is always surrounded by pieces of brain cell, and most of them are deteriorating.

Why is all this going on in the brain? Are the molecules to blame? Why have the brain particles clustered around the plaques? Alois Alzheimer didn't know in 1906. Eighty years later, there is still uncertainty.

And those neurofibrillary tangles, those intertwined wool-like fibres that Alzheimer noticed, what has caused them? Under the microscope, they could also be described as coils, like springs on a bed. These same lesions are found in the brains of people with Parkinson's disease when it has affected the brain area, and in adults with Down's syndrome. Interestingly, similar tangles have been found in the brains of boxers suffering punch-drunk symptoms. Scientists are, not surprisingly, baffled by the appearance of these tangles in so many different types of people. The causes of their lesions are varied: the Parkinson's disease sufferer is often a victim of a virus, the person with Down's syndrome is retarded because of a genetic fault, and the boxer's brain has received a traumatic shaking. What, then, has brought about the tangles in the brain of an Alzheimer sufferer who has caught no germ, had a normal birth and has received no blows to the head?

As if the tangles and plaques aren't enough to change the characteristics of the brain, scientists have also noted what they refer to as 'granulovacuolar changes'. Cells in the memory-storing hippocampus region become filled with fluid and a granular or grain-like material. What this grainy substance is doing in the brain of an Alzheimer sufferer raises another question. Certainly, as the grain grows, mental functions decrease.

There are two other noticeable changes in an Alzheimer brain. In some of the vessels, amyloid (found at the core of the plaques) has been discovered breaking in, so to speak, to the vessel wall. Just what the significance of the amyloid is here is another mystery, but it could signify an abnormality in the immune system of the brain.

The fifth change in the brain structure is the presence of what are known as Hirano bodies. These bodies, also found in the hippocampus region, are thought to encase vital granules which are responsible for bringing together proteins. Trapped in these Hirano bodies, the granules — known as ribosomes — cannot do their work and so memories cannot form.

Confusing as all these changes in the brain are, there is now little or no dispute that the lesions in an Alzheimer brain are directly related to the loss of mental and, following on from that, physical faculties. In Britain in 1968, epidemic experts conducted a post-mortem study of the brains and examined the medical records of 104 elderly patients and concluded once and for all that the more plaques and tangles found in the brain, the greater the loss of mental function. Swiss researchers, meanwhile, came up with the finding that there is a greater memory loss with a large concentration of plaques and tangles around the hippocampus. In the Swiss studies, the brains of 650 patients were studied, and every one with a high concentration of lesions suffered memory loss, whereas only 30 per cent of those with no lesions had amnesia.

The shrunken brain that Alzheimer found in his patient surprised him, and similar atrophy showing up on electronic scans within the skulls of people in their forties and fifies today would also be cause for alarm. However, it has been established that great shrinkage is not always obvious in Alzheimer's disease, particularly among the elderly. Further, the amount of any shrinkage is not always consistent with particular symptoms; if one person loses a quarter of his brain weight, say, he will not necessarily lose his speech, whereas another person might. Why doesn't the brain shrink in every case of Alzheimer's disease? If the cells die, why doesn't the brain always collapse inwards? Brain experts suggest that the disease process may lead to the growth of supporting brain tissue, but not new cells. The new tissue would help to maintain the size and weight of the brain.

However, if Alzheimer's disease strikes a 'young' person, a shrunken brain is usually found. The US Department of Health and Human Services describes the case of a 50-year-old woman whose brain was found to have atrophied alarmingly. What had happened to her had happened to Alzheimer's 51-year-old patient. The American woman was an attractive, pleasantly dressed, well-spoken woman, a former music teacher and pianist who, because of a fading memory, could no longer read music at sight. She just couldn't remember what a certain symbol meant. Her family said that for some time she had been having trouble taking telephone messages and remembering people. She could no longer look after the family accounts, and she had become lost on more than one occasion while driving. She knew she had a memory problem, yet when asked by a neurologist about her life, she was generally articulate and alert. She was asked a few everyday questions.

'Who is the President of the United States?'

'Reagan.'

'What's today's date?'

She scratched her head and smiled embarrassedly. 'Don't know.'

'The month?'

'Maybe April?' It was June.

'What year?'

'19 ... something.'

At one point she was asked to memorise three short phrases: red shoes, black box, 300 Broadway. She repeated the phrases, and the specialist went on to ask her to spell some common words such as 'world' and 'home' forwards and backwards. She was also asked to count down from 100 to 80. She ran into difficulties with all these tasks. Suddenly, the doctor asked her to repeat the phrases she had just learned.

'Red ...' That was all she could remember.

Until her failings in that typical exam to determine her mental status, the woman's appearance, mood and behaviour had not suggested that she might be suffering from a serious brain disease. The results of extensive physical and laboratory tests were largely negative. But X-rays with specialised equipment showed neurologists what they expected. The woman's brain showed widespread loss of nerve tissue in the cortex. The channels that circulate cerebral spinal fluid in the brain were also enlarged, another indication that brain substance had been lost and fluid had filled the gap. Despite the woman's ability to pass herself off as a 'normal' person, apart from some general vagueness, the X-rays gave away the fact that she was heading for serious mental impairment. She would never again be able to read music.

This woman's vagueness and memory loss was a clue that something might be amiss. Forgetfulness, like failing to turn off the gas or being unable to find the way home, might be other warning signs.

Signs for panic? Signs that Alzheimer's disease has struck? Not necessarily. A forgetful person might have dementia, but it might not be of the irreversible Alzheimer type.

3

Understanding dementia

Dementia, if classified as irreversible, is an insidious unrelenting force that ravishes the brain cells and hurtles the body onwards towards the grave. 'For family members, watching a loved one become increasingly deprived of his or her mental capacities is agonising,' says neurologist Miriam K. Aronson of New York's Albert Einstein College of Medicine.

Dementia is a name used to describe any one of a variety of problems that can occur within the brain. Anyone who begins to behave 'peculiarly', who shows a decline in his or her usual mental faculties, is suspected of dementing. The condition has nothing to do with those who are born with mental problems; the changes have to occur in a person who has behaved 'normally'. Dementia has been newly defined by the American Psychiatric Association as a syndrome characterised by a decline in previously acquired educational, occupational or social capabilities. Differences in behaviour can include forgetfulness, confusion, a change in emotion or the loss of ability to control toilet functions.

Dr R.L. Symonds, consultant psychiatrist at Oakwood Hospital, Maidstone, Kent, says of dementia: 'It is a deterioration of intellect so that the power of creative and intelligent thought is progressively diminished.' But he adds that it is 'not merely a diminution of intellect but a dissolution of the self... Dementia is a dismantling of the human being, starting at the most organised and complex part and proceeding with the failure of the central nervous system components. It involves brain cell death; it progressively involves lower parts of the central nervous system, so that if no other illnesses were to supervene, it would cause death.

It follows that dementia is a form of dying'.

There is not a kind word that can be said about it. Dr Carl Eisdorfer and Dr Donna Cohen, prominent psychiatrists from the University of Washington's Department of Psychiatry and Behavioural Sciences, comment: 'Dementing illness is a significant clinical problem, not only because of its devastating effect on the health and quality of life of the patient and family but also because of its malignancy and prevalence and its consequent social and economic impact upon society at large.'

Physical sickness and acute disease are socially acceptable. But mental disorders carry a stigma and are seen by some as being close to criminal. The ancient Greeks and Romans so feared the advancing years and the 'peculiarities' of growing old, that they looked on ageing as a disease.

Modern neuroscientists concede that the brain undergoes changes as it ages, but these do not have any serious effect on mental vigour. Picasso was still painting at 91, Toscanini still conducting at 89. Yet old age and the problems associated with it become an increasing cause of concern for many as they approach it. In today's youth-oriented society, the aged, particularly the aged infirm, are regarded as an increasing burden on society and governments. It is no wonder, then, that the moment someone is seen to have a slight memory impairment, he or she is held to be at the start of a downhill slide into senile retirement.

Of course, many alterations do occur as we age. Gathered together, our anticipated defects are daunting: thinning skin, loss of height, declining muscle strength, hardening of blood vessels, loss of lung elasticity, shrinkage of gums resulting in teeth loss, gastrointestinal problems, changed liver metabolism, kidney changes, weakened pelvic muscles, diminished reflexes, decreased taste and smell, deterioration of sight and hearing, a changed sleep pattern perhaps resulting in insomnia, and reduced brain weight. All these changes are part of the normal process of ageing.

When we're young, in our teens, old age is a million light years away. It's something we don't really think of. Dr Cees van Tiggelen, a Dutch psychogeriatrician working in Australia, says that in today's society old age is more of a cultural shock than for former generations. 'Time was when the old were looked up to for their wisdom and held an honoured place in society. The materialism of this industrial age soon stopped that. Now old is obsolete. Because society now has low expectations of the elderly, many tend to withdraw into "learned helplessness". This only increases the degenerative process because without the strains of life the coping capacity goes downhill rapidly. The physical possibilities of being active and participating in everything decreases. So, too, do the social and cultural possibilities of participating fully in everything.'

Another worker dealing with the aged says: 'People generally are a little prejudiced against the elderly. They are impatient with their slowness. They laugh at them because they do things they think are silly. As we age and our parents age we become irritated because they tend to misplace things and can't see or hear so well. Then they have difficulty walking and we find we have to drive them around or run errands. They forget things, forget the names of friends, and you might think what a terrible thing it is to become old and lose your memory like that. As we grow older the years seem to pass more quickly than when we were children, and we are aware that we are being catapulted towards that very time that we dreaded.'

Through the centuries, contrary to beliefs that among certain races the elderly were held in esteem, they were often considered as troublesome and dealt with accordingly. The Hunzakuts, who live on the border between Pakistan and China and between Afghanistan and Russia, required in the nineteenth century the eldest son to place his old parents in a conical basket, transport them to the mountain tops, and cast them over. And after battles with the British towards the end of the century, elderly men were chosen as envoys to deal with the victors because they were seen as expendable if anyone became trigger-happy.

We might wonder as we age whether we will lose our memory, become confused or bedridden. Certainly with age comes some loss. Two American researchers, R.L. Kane and R.A. Kane, who visited six countries, concluded: 'Nowhere are the processes of old age preventable — the elderly in all the countries studied experienced losses in power, functional ability, memory and mental faculties, friendships and social roles.'

However, researchers now say that, contrary to earlier beliefs, certain crucial parts of the brain do not fade away with old age among people who are in good health. They believe that although some other aspects of the intellect do diminish, the decline is slight. Some of the most important forms of intellectual growth, researchers around the world now agree, can continue well into the eighties. Declines in intelligence can be reversed in some cases because the causes are brought on by symptoms that can be treated and result in stress being removed from the mind. Countless numbers of people who had led vigorous lives might have ended their days in mental institutions unnecessarily, just because their mental problems were not properly understood. And once the mind stops working it can carry the body towards death. What does distinguish normal ageing, normal deterioration of the brain, from dementia? According to one expert in the field of dementia, Professor Michael Hall of England's Southampton University, there is no clear-cut line between mental impairment and the normal ageing process. Researchers have found that some of the lesions found in an Alzheimer brain, such as plaques and tangles, occur to some extent in the normal process of ageing. Losing one's short-term memory, adopting a more conservative attitude to life, along with a desire to live in the past, are well-known changes with maturing and age.

Yet, says Professor Hall, harmless senile forgetfulness may well be an early form of senile dementia, and while such features normally remain within acceptable limits, they might 'cross the line' to the point where the person's ability to live alone is impaired.

Sometimes this decline is brought on by the person himself, encouraged by the expectations of those around him. Both the person and his relatives might believe that old age brings an unavoidable mental deterioration. Warner Schaie, an eminent researcher on ageing, says: 'The expectation of a decline is a self-fulfilling prophecy. Those who don't accept the stereotype of a helpless old age, but instead feel they can do as well in old age as they have at other times in their lives, don't become ineffective before their time.'

Within the past five years, researchers have found that one key mental faculty — 'crystallised intelligence' is what they call it — continues to rise during the life span of active people who remain in good health and free from strokes. Researchers describe this crystallised intelligence as the ability to use an accumulated body of general information to make judgements. We use it to understand debates, to follow the cases put in newspaper editorials, or to find solutions to difficult problems. Much of the research into this intelligence has been carried out by John Horn, a psychologist at the University of Denver, who says the ability to bring to mind and entertain many different facets of information improves in many people over their vital years. This shows up in the ability of older people to speak more eloquently with rich, evocative fluency. 'They can say the same thing in five different ways. In our research, they're better in this sort of knowledge than the young people we see,' says Horn.

Scientists also refer to 'fluid intelligence', a set of abilities involved in seeing and using abstract relationships and patterns. Generals use this intelligence when trying to work out which moves the enemy will make before sending their own soldiers into battle; we use it when playing chess or writing a fictitious short story. Dr Horn concedes that fluid intelligence declines from early adulthood onwards, and he finds support in this theory from Martha Storandt, a psychologist at Washington University. But, she says, although the decline of fluid intelligence has some impact, people learn to compensate, even in later life. 'You can still learn what you want to,' she says. 'It's just that it takes a little longer.'

Studies show that if there are any setbacks in the healthy ageing brain, they are more of a nuisance than a major problem — such as not being able to recall names or remember telephone numbers. In general, though, knowledge increases with age, a fact discovered by researchers Roy and Janet Lachman who conducted a series of tests at the University of Houston. They found that knowledge about the names of world leaders, the capitals of countries, the signs of danger in the streets, increased with age through the seventies. The oldest group they tested was more efficient in recalling general facts than people of middle age or in their twenties.

Some medical scientists suggest that the developing human brain acquires more cells than it will ever need, and no matter how much 'normal' loss there might be, there are plenty of surviving cells to allow a person to think clearly.

Professor Hall of Southampton University is in agreement with experts around the world that the speed and the extent to which a personality disintegrates varies considerably; and, he says, those most severely affected experience not only a diminished capacity for simple everyday tasks so that they cannot survive without considerable assistance, but they invariably face a shortened life expectancy. An ageing person and a younger victim of Alzheimer's disease, then, could be seen to be travelling down the same confused road.

Dr Symonds of Maidstone's Oakwood Hospital sees these demented travellers as time travellers — people who are returning to an earlier age of their lives. We do not know whether Alois Alzheimer's patient ever talked to him about the mid-1800s, but modern researchers have certainly come across many cases of people who go back in time.

'The effect of short-term memory disorder is profound and means that the person literally lives in the past because he cannot live in the present,' says Dr Symonds. 'This is not because he is neurotically fleeing from the present, preferring to remember the past, but because he does not have the apparatus to construe the world which is existing now. He does not receive it as clearly, understand it or store it as well as his memories.' The expression 'second childhood', says the psychiatrist, is commonly used for the aged person and is certainly true for the person with advanced dementia who sees himself living as a child with his parents, yet troubled by the 'intruding phantoms' of the present, who are in fact his own children.

That those afflicted return to their earlier years is clearly indicated in elderly migrants living in Melbourne, Australia, a city with a large ethnic community. As Alzheimer's disease progresses, their command of the English they learned on arrival in Australia 40 or 50 years earlier diminishes, and they revert to their mother language to the point where they no longer understand questions asked in English. One woman, born in Italy, says: 'It is very difficult for our grandchildren who are now second-generation Australians and can only understand a little Italian. My husband talks only in the language he knew years ago. It is the only way I can talk to him, but even then he does not always understand me. He talks about Naples where he grew up as a boy, and I think sometimes he believes he is there, but not in the right house. He keeps going away down the road looking for the house he used to live in.'

G.K. Wilcock, consultant physician in geriatrics and general medicine at Oxford's Radcliffe Infirmary, agrees that the mental changes that occur as part of the normal ageing process include impaired short-term memory, the adoption of a more conservative outlook on life, a tendency to be more rigid and inflexible and a pessimistic outlook 'coupled in many cases with a desire to return to the good old days, which in reality were often anything but good'.

Mr Wilcock adds: 'In normal, elderly people, this makes no inroad into their ability to live an independent existence. The normal psychological changes of ageing are not a bar to adequate intellectual functioning, and many well-known people have produced great works in their latter years including Somerset Maugham, Picasso and Bertrand Russell.' He points out, however, that if the psychological changes begin to affect day-to-day existence, something abnormal might be happening. It is difficult to define the changes in 'normal' ageing, he says, because there is an overlap between normal and diseased conditions in the elderly. It is generally accepted, though, that with advancing years there is loss in brain weight and, along with other losses, the appearance of plaques and neurofibrillary tangles, mainly in the hippocampus area.

In fact, the brain might shrink by as much as 20 to 30 per cent between the ages 25 and 70. Yet even with an atrophied brain a 70-year-old can remain mentally alert. There is nothing we can do about the loss of our brain cells over the course of our lives, a loss that can be as much as a half. And we can all expect to develop some plaques and tangles.

'Some decline of mental function can be anticipated with ageing,' says Dr Marsel Mesulam, a Boston neurologist, 'but experience and wisdom can prevail.'

Dementia attacks the brain in different ways — at least that is what the various names given for it would have us believe. It is described as 'senility', 'senile dementia', 'pre-senile dementia', 'chronic brain syndrome', 'multi-infarct disease' and 'Alzheimer's disease'. It also used to be known as 'hardening of the arteries', which is inaccurate. In 1956, the United States National Institute of Mental Health questioned the then popular conception that mental problems among the elderly were inevitable, resulting from a hardening of the arteries in the brain. Using a system that enabled an average blood flow to be read, researchers found that the average supply of blood and oxygen to the brain in healthy elderly volunteers was not much less than in healthy people many years younger.

Dementia simply means that mental faculties have been impaired or greatly reduced — or in many cases removed altogether. When someone is demented they are not crazy or psychopathic. They have simply lost the ability to function in a way we all accept as normal. You see the effect when there is a decline of intellect and a change in behaviour and personality. In most cases, dementia results from progressive shrinking of the brain; but what causes this is still unknown. The condition is called pre-senile dementia when it happens to people below the age of 65 and senile dementia in older men and women. Neuroscientists — those who study the brain — have established that the disorders causing dementia belong to a group of brain diseases that share certain features. Certainly in every case the disease involves the accelerated death of nerve cells. Most times it is a selective death. Scientists and pathologists have found that the disease attacks a particular type of nerve cell or several kinds of cell confined to a particular area of the nervous system. Why are these cells assaulted? That is what researchers are trying to find out. They have come up with some answers, answers that show that chemical factors are behind the problem, or infections or a breakdown in the immune system.

Dementia can be caused by different diseases, the most frequent and irreversible being Alzheimer's. The second most common type of untreatable dementia, affecting between 12 and 20 per cent of those with dementia, is multi-infarct dementia, brought about by a series of strokes within the brain.

Small though these strokes may be, they whittle away at the brain tissue to the extent that they impair memory and the ability to think logically. The effect is rather like applying a series of tourniquets and forgetting to release them. Starved of blood, the areas beyond the restricted parts die. Because the damage is patchy, the course of the illness fluctuates with each small stroke. The tiny clots of blood that form cause the destruction.

Mr S.G.P. Webster, consultant geriatrician at the Chesterton Hospital, Cambridge, explains that during post-mortem examinations of the brain, small areas of injury caused by minute haemorrhages can be seen.

'The majority of elderly people are not demented. Many will be troubled by benign forgetfulness, but only 10 per cent will suffer from significant dementia,' says Mr Webster. 'Like most undesirable conditions, dementia rises in frequency with increasing **age**, so that its incidence in the over-eighties reaches 20 per cent. About one quarter of cases are due to cerebral destruction caused by vascular disease... In more than twice as many patients the reason for the cerebral shrinkage is not so obvious. These are often described as examples of senile or Alzheimer type dementia. Alzheimer initially described this form of mental deterioration in young patients, but this picture of pre-senile dementia is now thought to be identical to that most commonly found in the elderly.'

The geriatrician explains that on detailed microscopic examination of the cerebral cortex, many abnormalities — those neurofibrillary tangles and senile plaques, in particular — will be found among the brain cells. These features, though, are not found exclusively in the brains of demented patients. Examples will be present in most elderly patients, but the quantity is markedly increased in patients previously known to have been demented.

Multi-infarct dementia can sometimes be mistaken for Alzheimer's disease because the damage to the brain affects speech, memory and the ability to control movement. However, an examination of the history of the affected person usually provides the clues. If the man or woman suddenly behaves strangely, it is usually a sign that a series of small strokes have occurred; Alzheimer's disease, on the other hand, creeps in, so that odd behaviour does not instantly begin. Multi-infarct dementia usually appears between the ages of 40 and 60; Alzheimer's disease usually manifests itself beyond the age of 65, although for some unknown reason a growing number of people seem to be falling victim to the disease at a much earlier age.

In most cases, those with multi-infarct dementia have a history of high blood pressure, vascular disease or previous strokes. The problem often occurs in just one part of the brain, so the symptoms are limited to a specific faculty, such as hand or leg movements or speech. Doctors refer to these infarcts as 'localised' symptoms, whereas the overall effects of Alzheimer's disease are known as 'global' symptoms.

Beyond the initial point of change — a sudden switch in behaviour — multi-infarct sufferers might then start to display all the symptoms of someone affected by Alzheimer's disease. But this deterioration can be stopped if further strokes can be prevented. Stopped, but not reversed. What brain cells a person loses are lost for ever.

So there is the Alzheimer type of dementia, and there is multi-infarct dementia, neither of which is reversible. There is a third dementia class, a miscellaneous group which includes both treatable and untreatable conditions. Progressive and dementing brain diseases that are less common than Alzheimer's and multi-infarct dementias are multiple sclerosis, Parkinson's disease, Huntington's disease, Pick's disease and Creutzfeldt-Jakob disease.

Multiple sclerosis is one of the more well-known neurological diseases. It is characterised by the progressive destruction of the insulating material covering the nerve fibres. The disease's progress is an 'up and down' affair, but its conclusion is usually a deterioration of mental and physical faculties.

Parkinson's disease strikes older people and brings on tremors throughout the body. Drugs help, but so far nothing has been found to halt the progression of the disease. In advanced cases, symptoms of dementia can appear.

Symptoms of Huntington's disease start to show in early middle age and can include a change in personality and mental decline. 'Flickering' of the face, restlessness and, in more advanced cases, severe uncontrollable flailing of limbs, head and body follow. Mental faculties can fall away into dementia. One of the frightening things about this disease is that children with a parent suffering from it have a 50 per cent chance of inheriting it themselves.

Pick's disease symptoms are similar to those of Alzheimer's disease. However, it is a different malady because changes in the brain tissue are not the same.

Creutzfeldt-Jakob disease is caused by one of several infectious agents and can lead to dementia. A virus, lying dormant in the body for years, becomes activated and brings about a rapidly progressing dementia accompanied by a change in gait and by muscle spasms.

Sometimes, medical problems are wrongly diagnosed as being senile dementia when in many cases they are reversible. Delirium, for example, is sometime: confused with dementia in older people. This is because it can make someone confused or forgetful or behave inappropriately. The term 'delirium' is now used by most workers to cover quietly delirious people as well as the more agitated who behave in a way most of us expect when we think of 'delirium'. Its literal translation from the Latin is to rave, be deranged, go out of the furrow when ploughing.

Another condition that could result in loss of memory or confusion and bring on temporary dementia is depression. As long ago as 1961, a specialist emphasised that old people suffering from depression are at particular risk of being labelled as demented. Professor Tom Arie, a specialist in health care of the elderly and who is attached to Britain's University of Nottingham, points out that several recent reports have shown that 10 to 20 per cent of patients who are examined for dementia turn out to have other disorders.

When depression is the cause, it is understandable why, at first, it leads to a wrong assessment. For a large number of older people, depression is a reaction to losses: retirement from a loved job, bereavement, ill health, loneliness, poverty. Mr Tony Whitehead, a British psychiatrist, says: 'The individual who is depressed feels miserable and unhappy all the time, with a worsening at certain times of the day. There is often a slowing up of thought and actions... The appetite is usually lost, with little being eaten or drunk, and sleep is inevitably disturbed.'

The type of depression commonly misdiagnosed as dementia is the so-called 'endogenous depression' which can eventually result in a much more severe impairment of general functions — the sufferer may become quite mute, for instance.

A study of Alzheimer's disease sufferers carried out at the Albert Einstein College of Medicine, New York, revealed that demented patients were found to exhibit a high prevalence of depressed moods as well as disturbances in sleep and appetite, problems in concentrating, loss of interest and an inability to experience pleasure. In effect, some unfortunate people suffer from depression as a *secondary* problem to Alzheimer's disease. Three psychiatrists from the Albert Einstein College, Ira Katz, Miriam Aronson and Rochelle Lipkowitz, suggest that some of the apathy and withdrawal found in some people with dementia might be caused by what is known as retarded depression, whereas the hyperactivity, irritability and aggression found in others might be the result of agitated depression. Sometimes this secondary depression responds to treatment with antidepressants. In other words, an Alzheimer sufferer can undergo a change of character for the better as long as he or she has depression secondary to dementia. Antidepressants will help the person's mood, but they will not help the disease.

Professor Aronson says that for victims of dementia, the losses are, at the beginning, emotionally painful. 'It is not surprising, therefore, that depression often co-exists with dementia,' she says. This was found in 20 per cent of a group of people studied. Other researchers have been shocked to learn that 20 per cent of the elderly population suffer from depression.

Along with delirium and depression are several other organic brain syndromes that cause problems similar to those of senile dementia but which might be reversible. These can be brought about by trauma resulting from a severe blow to the head, or even relatively minor head injuries if elderly. What usually happens in these cases is that bleeding within the brain results in blood collecting between the skull and the brain, putting pressure on the cells and damaging them. Infections that can be caused by a virus or fungus are also to blame, as are nutritional deficiencies. Nutritional problems are often found with elderly people, particularly those living alone. A pensioner not eating properly may show mental symptoms before physical ones; lack of the B vitamins, for example, might bring on depression, irritability and forms of amnesia. Another nutritional problem is lack of blood sugar — if there is not enough in the bloodstream, confusion and a change in personality might result.

The side effects of drugs, excessive alcohol and toxins such as carbon monoxide are obvious causes of brain impairment. Circulatory problems precipitating heart complaints and strokes are also causes of disorders of the brain; a condition known as transient ischaemic attack, caused by a poor supply of blood to the brain, results in difficulty in speaking, dizziness and nausea. These symptoms last only a few minutes or hours, but such attacks could be advanced warnings that a major stroke is pending.

Neurological symptoms resulting from an excessive amount of fluid surrounding the brain and any type of growth or tumour inside the skull also have serious effects.

As well as these organic syndromes, a number of psychiatric problems can be confused with senile dementia. Depression, talked about earlier, can be so severe that it appears identical to senile dementia. This 'pseudodementia', like many other cases of organic brain syndromes, can be reversed unless ignored for so long that the person goes into a permanent state of 'hibernation'.

Basically, pseudodementias all show a characteristic loss of memory. This is not restricted to the elderly — it does develop in younger people who suffer from depression. In the young, who might have lost a job or a parent or failed an exam, depression can cause amnesia. But in the elderly, depression can precipitate such a severe memory loss that something more serious might be suspected. Usually, this follows some form of bereavement such as death of a partner, retirement, a change in finances or moving from a familiar environment. In many cases, these memory losses are temporary. Sometimes they are exaggerated by the very medicines

that are given to aid memory. One of the problems is that the elderly do not absorb drugs so easily from the intestinal tract, and their
kidneys and livers are less efficient. Consequently, their brains are
under a two-pronged assault: the depressed elderly person is
already in danger of some memory lapse, and then the drugs work
against him. One survey of patients in Massachusetts nursing
homes showed that 25 per cent had senile symptoms that were
treatable or preventable. The symptoms were brought on by
thyroid disorders, vitamin B_{12} deficiency and the side effects of
drugs. US researchers have found that uncontrolled and improper
drug use by the elderly in their own homes in the hope of con-
trolling heart rhythms or aiding sleep can cause confusion, blurred
vision and the symptoms of dementia. The brain of an older person
is more sensitive to anti-anxiety drugs such as diazepam (Valium)
and chlordiazepoxide (Librium) and as a result the taker suffers
lethargy and confusion.

Sometimes the elderly have wrong impressions about their own
conditions. They *think* they are severely losing their memories, but
some 75 per cent of those examined are found to have normal recall
for their age. They might not have the efficient memories of youth,
but there is nothing more to suggest they have dementia.

Scientists around the world refer to Alzheimer's disease as 'senile
dementia'. Dementia, of course, is an illness which affects the ability to think clearly and coordinate the body's movements. Senility
does *not* mean dementia; its interpretation, from a Latin root, is
'old'. It is not a medical term and has no agreed meaning in scientific circles. However, it is a commonly used word — a 'catchall
term' is how one psychiatrist describes it — that implies disturbances in the thinking processes of the elderly. The word is often
used to describe vague concepts about changes, particularly memory changes, in later life.

Dr Kenneth Sakauye, chief of Geriatric Psychiatry at Michael
Reese Hospital, Chicago, says 'senility' is caused by vascular disease, like strokes, or an increase in brain pressure, a theory not
widely endorsed. Sakauye says pressure occurs when the brain produces more of the fluid that surrounds it than it can reabsorb.
Chronic drug and alcohol abuse, more prevalent among the elderly
than generally thought, can also contribute to senility, he says.

'There are also drug toxic effects — that is, the effects of medicines taken by the elderly. Depression is another major cause of

intellectual disturbances. There are other multiple causes, related to many kinds of illnesses. There are 30 to 50 types of diseases that can result in brain dysfunction, aside from Alzheimer's.'

Dr Sakauye gives his version of what happens to the mind when senility occurs: 'With Alzheimer's disease, the usual thing that happens is atrophy of the brain. Cells beginning to die are replaced by another type of tissue that has a characteristic cell pattern. The onset of Alzheimer's tends to be generally a very slow process. One doesn't notice a clear date of onset. It has been developing in people in their fifties. The later the process occurs, the milder the affliction.

'Senility caused by drug and alcohol abuse is also a matter of destroying brain cells. And in the case of a vascular disease, blood is shut off to the brain. For instance, there can be small strokes in the area of the brain related to intellectual functions that do not necessarily affect motor functions (for example, movement of arms and legs). In this instance, there is generally evidence of blood vessel disease elsewhere in the body.'

Senility, then, if we accept its popular interpretation as meaning that something is amiss in the brain, is not a normal process of growing old. America's National Institute on Ageing emphasises that although 'senility' is something most of us fear, we are not all likely to fall victim to it as we advance in years. Senility, says the Institute, is the word commonly used to describe a large number of conditions with an equally large number of causes, many of which respond to treatment. The symptoms of what is popularly called 'senility', the Institute points out, include serious forgetfulness, confusion, and certain other changes in personality and behaviour. Whereas doctors and their patients once routinely dismissed these symptoms as incurable effects of old age, it is now accepted that this is not necessarily so. Small lapses in memory in old age do not signify senility, either. If there is slight confusion or occasional forgetfulness throughout life, it may signify only 'an overload of facts in the brain's storehouse of information'.

Many memory changes are temporary, like those that follow the death of a loved one or during a stressful situation that makes concentration difficult. Older people are often accused of losing their memory — they blame themselves sometimes, too — when in fact it is not really happening. Look at a younger person who does something absent-minded such as locking the keys in the car or forgetting to turn off the gas; this person is never accused of 'going senile'. Yet, interestingly, the mind of a 60-year-old can often be sharper than that of someone aged 30 to 40. As described previously, studies on intelligence in later life have shown that healthy people who remain intellectually active retain alert minds to the ends of their lives. This fact is in contrast to earlier studies which left researchers with the conclusion that intelligence declines with age. Tests have shown that the healthy aged brain works as hard and efficiently as a healthy young one. The majority of people retain, and in some cases raise, their intellectual competence as they age.

While Dr Sakauye says there are up to 50 types of diseases that can bring about problems in the brain, the Institute on Ageing believes some 100 reversible conditions could mimic mental disorders. A minor head injury, a high fever, an adverse reaction to drugs or poor nutrition can all temporarily upset the normal activity of sensitive brain cells. If left untreated, these conditions can result in permanent brain damage and even death.

From the age of twenty we lose some 50 000 nerve cells every day, which may, or may not, be responsible for intellectual decline in old age. Despite this loss, says Robert Butler of the Mount Sinai School of Medicine, at least some parts of the brain continue to grow as long as a person lives. This growth, he explains, can be seen in the dendrites, the branchlike extensions through which the cell body receives virtually all messages from cells in other parts of the body.

'Perhaps at some point,' he says, 'the brain cells that are regressing and dying begin to outnumber the cells that are surviving and growing, but it is encouraging to note that the brain seems to have a unique built-in protective mechanism that allows it to compensate for the loss of some of its cells over time.'

Butler says that if there appear to be increased intellectual problems, particularly memory problems, as a person ages, they may be due to difficulties in acquiring new information, storing it away with all the learned material of a lifetime, or retrieving it quickly. Difficulties in acquiring new information may be caused or aggravated by visual or hearing problems. A person suffering from the common age-related loss of ability to hear high-frequency sounds may have problems hearing human voices or interpreting speech. Failing concentration or lack of motivation can also prevent proper registration of new information.

'The ability to store information may be compromised by increasing susceptibility to the effects of interference,' Butler speculates. 'The older central processing system seems less able to handle the overload of stimuli created by the thousands of messages the body receives every minute. As a result, information can be pushed aside by newer incoming information. Reaction speed is one aspect of intelligence that may indeed decrease with age. Therefore, even if information is properly acquired and stored, an older person might be slower in searching for, recovering, and producing that information from memory. It is reassuring, however, that none of these age-related changes appears to be insurmountable until extreme old age. Older people often compensate for benign forms of memory loss by keeping notes, establishing routines and planning ahead.'

For those who are diagnosed as having 'real' dementia, they face a strange form of dying, says Dr Symonds of Maidstone. 'It is an awe-inspiring illness ... it deserves to some extent the description of second childhood. As a personal illness it is a strange form of dying. Rather than being aware that one is losing the functions of a number of organs through illness, one's organ of awareness is itself affected. How does this affect the person?

'An adult human being might wish, in the early stages of his dying, to compose himself to meet and live through this final part of his life, to carry out the emotional work of dying. The person with dementia is, however, unable to do his dying for himself, as he cannot experience it as a fully competent human being ... Obviously, the loss of intellectual ability is appreciated by the remainder of the intellect. Many dementing patients appreciate their deterioration and some will even be able to describe it. A common concern that may take them to their doctor is that their mental sluggishness is more than might be expected from age alone, although many will take refuge in the idea of old age.'

Dr Symonds says that with the sluggishness comes sadness for the mental life the affected person used to have, a memory of acuteness and mental ability. The sadness that overwhelms the person is the sort that resembles grief for a dead relative. Just as in bereavement grief can be coped with better if discussed with an empathetic listener, so this sadness is helped by talk. A reminiscence of previous achievements will also aid the retention of dignity. To his acquaintances, a dementing man is still a living memorial to the person he was. If they realise this aspect of dementia, friends and relatives can react with mourning, which can be carried out in advance of the final biological death and relieve the grief that does occur when the person eventually dies.

With poor intellectual grasp, poor memory and other specific disabilities, the dementing person becomes disorientated. He loses a sense of familiarity with the environment and becomes unaware of events taking place in the world. Dr Symonds has found that dementia initially hardens the personality and brings out the salient features of what the person always had. It is likely that aggression, paranoia and the self-blaming aspects of depression were in the personality before dementia crept in.

Whatever the individual symptoms, doctors and health care workers are painfully aware that unless a breakthrough is found, dementia will be an even greater problem around the world within a decade. Professor P.H. Millard, an expert in geriatrics at St George's Hospital Medical School, London, observed in the *British Medical Journal* in 1981:

'The last scene of all is not inevitably Shakespeare's [description of] second childishness and mere oblivion, sans teeth, sans eyes, sans taste, sans everything; for the corollary of two demented people in every ten aged 80 and over is that eight out of ten are not demented. Nevertheless, the continuing age drift means that by 1988 a health district containing 250 000 people will have to provide services for 3000 elderly people with dementia; and health service planners are well aware that their major task in the next decade will be coping with organic mental impairment in the elderly...'

Another British expert in the field of geriatrics, Mr S. Luke, Consultant Psychogeriatrician at the Luton and Dunstable Hospital, says that the psychiatry of old age has until recently been a neglected area of work, both inside medical circles and in the world generally. 'Old age,' he says, 'has been considered synonymous with a general decline of physical and mental abilities. It is now recognised that as the number of people surviving into their 80s grows, the problems of management multiply and the importance of early diagnosis of both physical and psychiatric illness becomes even greater.'

4

The effects

I picture the cells in Mother's brain twinkling and fading out one by one, feeble stars on a vast horizon.

— *A daughter*

It attacks silently, stealthily. It wipes away smiles, dries up tears, makes a mockery of speech; it builds an impenetrable wall around the brain, bricking in emotions, cutting off communication. It becomes the puppet master, dangling its human dolls on an invisible thread. It gnaws relentlessly at the fuse box until, at long last, the lights go out.

Alzheimer's disease, British geriatrician Sir Martin Roth commented after post-mortem examinations of the brains of those who had succumbed, looks like death from boredom. It removes the capacity to read, converse, understand the story in a television show or follow the melody in a piece of music.

Because the neurofibrillary tangles and neuritic plaques develop so slowly, the effects on the brain and consequently on the mental and physical faculties are at first imperceptible. In the beginning, the memory goes, a loss that the person himself might be aware of before anyone else. A woman might return from the shops and find a saucepan has boiled dry because she left the gas on. It's one of those forgetful traits of human nature, something a neighbour did the week before, so it's no cause for concern. She'll chide herself for being silly, for 'almost burning the house down', and then it will pass from her mind. A few days later she might forget where she's put the car keys, and when she's found them she can't find the car. As the disease develops, even the ability to recognise forgetfulness is lost. Frequently an elderly person is unable to find the spectacles he has pushed up on his forehead. That's a harmless, perhaps eccen-

tric part of growing old. But with Alzheimer's disease, as geriatrician Richard Besdine of the Harvard Medical School points out,
you forget you ever had glasses.

As this forgetfulness continues, relatives begin to notice. Someone in the family will be unable to find a plate or a cushion,
perhaps, and the item will eventually be found out in the garden.
The story of Rita Young, once a beautiful model for the well-
known Australian artist Norman Lindsay, typifies the onset of the
disease. Her Eurasian features and fine figure adorn many of
Lindsay's paintings, which continue to bring enormous prices at
auctions around the world. Today, at the age of 64, Rita has
Alzheimer's disease. Her daughter, Marguerite Young, talks of her
mother so that others may understand the disease:

'Rita was always called "vague" by the family. She seemed content to drift into her own dream world, obviously useful for long
poses as a model. Consequently, the first of three stages of the disease, the "forgetfulness" phase, almost passed us by unnoticed. We
didn't realise anything was wrong with her until my father retired
in 1979. A move to a home on the New South Wales central coast
turned out to be less than blissful. Rita had looked forward to moving to a seaside-bushland setting, but she became disoriented in the
new house. She misplaced things and often couldn't complete simple tasks. My father, George, who did most of the cooking but
none of the cleaning, would despair when he couldn't find a kitchen
gadget. A can opener would be lost for days, although Rita would
swear she'd put it back on the kitchen shelf. Eventually George
would find it in the linen press or under the bed. When they retired
at night, George would often find alternating sheet, blanket, sheet,
blanket and no pillow slips. Dishes were washed without detergent.
Rita would eat sandwiches with a knife and fork. She would give
George tea when he asked for coffee. George, never known for his
patience, scolded her. Rita, who had always been accommodating
and serene, became anxious and fought back. They argued.

'George complained that Rita was lazy, neglectful of herself and
the house. Rita, in turn, complained that George was impatient and
self-centred. We were embarrassed. The tables had been turned —
they were the fighting children, and we were to be the mediating
parents. We didn't want to know and hoped desperately they
would solve their own problems. One evening, Rita threw a tantrum. She had never played cards with the family in nearly 40 years

of marriage. We laughed at her when she asked if she could play She let forth with a volley of abuse. We didn't care for her, she said, crying. Then she vomited. I felt vilified. My mother, who was normally so calm, was sick and it was time we acknowledged it ...'

As Marguerite notes, Alzheimer's disease tends to develop in phases. These cannot be rigidly defined because people react in different ways. The first phase, though, affects everyone. It seems innocuous enough: those occasional lapses of memory, a flattening of the personality, perhaps, or disinterest in a newspaper hardly ring the alarm bells. Sometimes the person will be more reserved with groups of people and will find more comfort when surrounded by relatives and close friends.

A Yorkshire woman says of her 66-year-old father: 'He was always a good conversationalist. He was on the committee of the Rugby club and was always popular at dinners. One year he forgot to go to the annual dinner, even though he was talking about it to one of the other officials on the telephone just a day earlier. Mum and I had gone out ourselves and when we returned home we were surprised that he was still there. When we asked why he hadn't gone, he said "Oh, was it tonight?" That was the start of it all, as far as I can recall. He lost interest completely in the club, yet it had been part of his life. He lost the ability to converse and just sat in his chair, not reading, not watching television. Just sitting there, you know?'

The early symptoms are more recognisable in some people than in others. An accountant who begins to make mistakes in calculations is noticed more than someone who never was a good mathematician and continues to make errors when adding up. Similarly, a good conversationist who begins to 'dry up' raises more comment from friends and relatives than a man or woman who was more of a listener. In most cases where there is a change in behaviour, loss of immediate memory is the root of the problem. The accountant will forget that 15 and 17 add up to 32; his mind will not recall a process that once came naturally. Others may forget the day or lose a sense of hours of the day, thinking it is morning when it is late afternoon. For those living alone, life becomes a danger to themselves and a nuisance to others. Many *are* in danger of burning the house down, because the stove is left on time after time.

Some specialists believe, however, that even those with fairly severe dementia can continue to live alone as long as they are able to maintain the habits of a lifetime. Every day may be identical, but the demented person will be content in his or her world. Any change could destroy this state. Such changes could be a move to a new house initiated by a friend or relative, different neighbours or visiting nurses — even a change in medication. Often it is the early stages of Alzheimer's disease or related disorders that are the most dangerous, when friends and relatives are not aware that something is going wrong.

'At first,' says an adviser on dementia, 'the sufferer shows no more than the forgetfulness often associated with advancing years, though it is more marked and disruptive. The memory becomes less and less reliable, but in a way that can deceive the casual acquaintance. Memories from the distant past may be well preserved but the injured brain cannot absorb fresh experience. By lunchtime, it is difficult to recall breakfast — fortunately not of itself a sign of dementia — and in extreme cases the period of a person's married life can be completely forgotten.'

It is impossible to follow the chemical processes that take part in the brain from the beginning, but clinical observations and the reports of relatives and friends are all in agreement that the early stages of the disease are minor changes in personality, social behaviour and intellectual functioning.

'My mother was always such a beautiful dresser,' says a woman in Los Angeles. 'She loved to dress up and go out to dinner. Even going to the local store was an occasion to brush her hair, put on a bit of make-up. Then she didn't seem to care about how she looked. They diagnosed Alzheimer's disease, and she just kept on going downhill and the only way we could get her to look nice was to do it for her ourselves.'

There are an endless number of stories that bring shudders to people who, through age or association or family, feel vulnerable and alarmed. The following is a Melbourne woman's story. Her husband is now 55. He has had the disease for three years.

'How could I fail to notice the moods, the selfishness, the ignorance of time-keeping in relation to other people and appointments. The quiet moving around the house. The disappearances to the furthest corner of the garden to clip bits off some insignificant little bush that didn't need pruning, when the bush near the back doorway was just about taking over the doorway. Disappearing to burn off rubbish in the incinerator, knowing that the smoke would invade the house and cause hay fever or asthma, but choosing not to remember that, as long as he could sneak away into his own little world away from decisions. The tying up of limbs of trees when they started to grow in the wrong direction and were getting in the way, instead of trimming them off, and doing this so often that in the end the trees were so trussed up that they began to strangle and overbalance.

'The picking over of garbage and burning off the burnable, instead of throwing it all out in the rubbish collection each week. This also allowed an excuse to light the incinerator and burn and poke and spend more time up the back of the yard away from the world of talk and decisions.

'Never being able to discuss something with my husband that just needed talking about, without it being turned around and fed back in the form of an argument. It was just a simple problem — why did it have to cause an argument?

'Why did I always feel like a school mistress when I asked that the simple things be done around the house that were a husband's part of the house-running? Why was I made to feel that it was my fault that the leaves were clogging the downpipes when it rained?

'The hours it took to put the holiday gear in the car, when all my husband had to do was carry the gear from the house and place it in the car. Why, if I hadn't finished packing one box, was this the one that he insisted had to go in first? What was wrong with all the others? Why was I made to feel that it was my fault he had to pack the car? After all, I had arranged the holiday, why didn't I pack the car also? In the end I did pack the car, because I could not stand by and watch this confused person practically fall apart because he had to make decisions about which box to put in first.

'The terrible confusion over whether the doors were locked or unlocked when we were going out. The number of times I have waited with front door key secretly poised in my hand, and then was forced to patiently wait while he stood in front of the door, fumbled for his keys in his pocket, select the key and finally open the door. His forward planning had completely disappeared, even on little things like opening doors.

'He never did learn how to change the stereo from radio to 'gram to tape. That required concentration. All he could manage was to turn over the record that was already selected, or turn the whole thing off if he thought you were out of ear-shot. But on the other hand, he always left every light on around the house wherever he went. Perhaps these were signs of insecurity that I didn't recognise at the time.

'Insisting that he only needed to shower every second day, but then not being able to remember whether this was shower day or not, getting cross when you told him it was shower day, and then forgetting to change to clean clothes when he did have a shower.

'Never calling me by name. Never thanking me for a well-thought-out, well-cooked meal. Not really knowing what he ate anyway, because he was watching TV during the meal... Having to be asked after 25 years of marriage whether or not I took milk in my tea. Not ever ringing friends or relations in an effort to keep in contact with them. Never writing home to the family in the UK.

'Never projecting and never making a decision. Working on the principle that if you don't make a decision, you can't make a mistake. No thought was ever given to how we paid the bills once he had given over his basic amount that contributed to the running of the household. The paying of bills was just left to providence and the little woman to work out. If he left things for long enough he knew that I would fix it, because I am like that.

'You try to help by taking him to all the people you can think of who might be able to calm him down, start him thinking of himself as a person, and try to get his brain stimulated with exercise, medication and anything else that may help. Of course, while you are doing all of this, you have to ignore the fact that you are being told that you are the one who is stopping him from driving the car, taking him to disagreeable people who are making him do exercises, making him take medication that he doesn't want to take, and letting people take blood from him.

'Within a few months, my husband was encouraged to start driving the car, and start a lawn-mowing round, with a lot of help from me. That also was not easy, because he had no idea which day to go to which area unless it was all written down. He didn't do any more than ten lawns a week, and that took him all week. He didn't get any money, but it kept him busy and out of the house talking to customers...

'The doctors he is now attending are hopeful that they may be able to reverse some of the damage with vitamins, diet and the correct antidepressant, and they also will maintain that the petrochemical atmosphere in the work situation contributed to his pre-senile dementia.

'Now we call it Alzheimer's disease. Whatever it is called, it is a very difficult condition to live with.'

There is no set pattern to the progression of the disease, but various symptoms appear. Following the initial memory losses, sufferers often begin to lose the ability to speak at their usual pace. But it really depends on which aspect of brain function is lost at first and fastest. Problems with language functions produce dysphasia in some sufferers; in others there may be interference with the organisation of body movements, producing dyspraxia. There are other possibilities. Many doctors disagree with a rigid notion of stages of dementia and of a definite type of deterioriation because relatives can be confused when their family member doesn't fit a pattern.

However, if a pattern can be typified, the formation of words is among the early difficulties. Hearing remains intact, but the ability to *understand* words begins to fade. Friends find themselves having to repeat a sentence because there is no response, or when there is it is not connected with what has already been said. It is as if the person is daydreaming. Of course, those with 'healthy' minds can be guilty of that, but when it happens often along with a slowing down of speech and a worsening memory, relatives begin to wonder if something is going wrong. The impaired person will deny there is any problem, and the more he is asked about it, the more irritable he becomes.

A Sydney woman's story: 'My husband was a clerk with a shipping company. They had to let him go from the job because he was making terrible mistakes. He would write out a letter in longhand for a secretary to type up and she wouldn't be able to understand it. Mike began to frighten me when he drove the car. He started to go through red lights, and the only way I could stop him driving was to hide the keys. He accused me of stealing them, which was quite true, but he also accused me of taking other things, which wasn't true. Then he started to get angry and frustrated. I asked him if he thought there was something wrong with his memory or if he was having headaches, and he told me not to be so bloody stupid. But I knew there was something wrong, and he finally agreed to come with me to a neurologist. He said Mike definitely had the symptoms of Alzheimer's disease and would only get worse.'

Another Australian woman says after her husband was diag-

nosed as having Alzheimer's disease: 'I had never heard of it and
was stunned at the implications. John had always been an extremely
active man, with a quick, intelligent, probing mind. I couldn't believe that already part of the brain had begun to "rot" and there was
no hope for a reversal. I was told that nothing could be done, and
that when he got worse, he could have to be committed. I vowed
that would never happen. I asked if there were any societies which
could help me to understand and to cope and was given the name of
one. When I telephoned, the doctor in charge said: "Mrs Field, it's
useless for you to come to me. All I can say to you is, God help you
and God bless you. No one can help!"'

At first, some men and women who start to lose control try to
conceal the problem. Even if they are unaware of Alzheimer's disease, they know something is happening and a lot of defence
mechanisms start to work all at once. They don't want to put
people out, be made a fuss of, and they don't like to envisage themselves as hospital cases. They don't like to admit either, that it —
whatever 'it' might be — is happening to them. To use a classic
expression: 'It's something that always happens to somebody else.'

During the first and much of the second stages, concealment of
the problem is often successful. A victim might write notes to remind himself to do a certain chore or to give instructions to a taxi
driver. 'Few people are anxious to admit their shortcomings,' says
Bob Browne, British adviser on the elderly, 'so it is not surprising
that dementia sufferers fabricate explanations to cover their lapses
of memory. New acquaintances are misidentified as relatives, and
residential homes become hotels or private houses and the like.
Making false statements to hide one's failing memory or lack of
understanding is called confabulation.'

Researchers have established that there is a great deal of 'confabulation' going on, because apart from not wishing to be a burden
on others or wanting to admit they have a problem, those who
realise they are losing their memories see the condition as a threat
to their independence. They try harder with the housework or the
office job or their factory work and insist that things are fine. And
they cling desperately to their memories. They talk about the past a
great deal, believing that it isn't all that far away, and when they
have such recall they convince themselves that their memories
aren't going after all. When suggestions are made that they *are*
losing their memories, they react with denials and, in some

cases, anger.

Sometimes it is difficult for a family to make an assessment. The affected person appears well physically, and may talk normally except for an occasional lapse. It's like trying to compare two drawings in a puzzle; they look identical, but minor changes have been made in one and you have to spot the difference. Some victims appear so normal that, far from trying to deny anything is wrong, they try to find out more about their problem. In a letter to a social worker in London a man wrote, in legible handwriting:

'My GP has recently informed my wife that I am suffering from Alzheimer's disease. As there is no address of a local contact on the leaflet which my wife obtained from him, I wonder if you could give me any advice or help in this matter. I would be glad to hear from you or I would be glad to be of any assistance ...'

There are no physical clues to an early-stage dementia sufferer. A Melbourne woman describes her mother:

'She has a beautiful chiselled face. Her hair is now white because she has stopped tinting it. Her smile never fails to turn her into a flirt ... She is a charmer and she is charmed by people, by nature, by life. I cherish those moments when she is charmed and charming.

'But my mother's mind is gone. Then it returns and goes again. She remembers nothing of the recent past. The more recent, the more instantly it is gone. Though her wit and humour and perceptiveness are astonishing. It is a frightening condition for one like me who has not dealt with minds beyond the ordinary.'

A Sydney man put this question to a specialist: 'My mother refuses to believe that there is anything wrong, and this causes dreadful arguments with the family, very ill husband and others. Her doctor has told us she has Alzheimer's disease, but will not tell her, knowing that she would be hostile to the fact. What can we do for help?'

He was told: 'No matter how you go about it, it's going to be a painful experience telling someone that her memory is going. Warmth, affection, a quiet place and a gentle approach are necessary. Perhaps it might be more acceptable coming from someone else other than you. After all, you are going to have to live with it every day, and it may be better that you are not blamed in some irrational way because you have broken the news. Then again, perhaps this may be a coward's way out? I have found it useful to explain that a part of the person is ageing more rapidly than the rest of him or her. That really it is a disease of memory but the rest is intact and there are ways of compensating for the loss of memory.'

The wife of a Melbourne academic, who started showing signs of dementia when he was just 49, says: 'At first, I put it down to his being an egghead. For ages, I thought I was just imagining it. Then it got to the stage when I knew something was wrong, but I didn't like to admit it. I suggested he see a doctor. I secretly thought he had had a stroke. He went and he said to the doctor: "I think something's happened to my neurons; my wife said to tell you." The doctor said: "Go home and tell your wife there's nothing wrong with you and to stop nagging." I was very upset about that, and for years I didn't go to a doctor about it because I knew there was something wrong and I wondered whether I was causing it. From that point on, until he got quite bad, he tried to cover it up so that no one suspected anything was wrong.'

Progression of Alzheimer's disease often involves a further loss of speech, confusion and disorientation. A British psychiatric nurse comments: 'The characteristic symptom of the confusional state is clouding of consciousness. This does not mean the person is drowsy — although he may be — but he cannot grasp the reality of his situation. He is unable to sustain attention and may behave in odd ways, drinking, for example, from a flower vase at the bedside.'

The affected person loses all track of time, does not know where he is, fails to recognise close relatives, wanders away from home and is unable to recall his own name and address. This distressing disorientation feature also encompasses new words, words that don't exist in the English language. This is a sign that the transmission system of the brain has seriously degenerated. There may be just the occasional strange word at first, but this onset of a new language is a warning of what is to come; speech will inevitably turn into meaningless babble.

Two US researchers at the University of Pennsylvania Hospital, Dr Myrna Schwartz and her associate Susan Williamson, have found certain groups of characteristics among Alzheimer patients. Some people, they have found, exhibit a decline in language abilities very early, yet others do not lose their speech until much later. The researchers have classified one language problem as a 'naming disorder.' In this group, a person repeats stereotype phrases or makes mistakes when using pronouns, referring to 'it' as 'she', or 'him' as 'you'. The afflicted man or woman might also not be specific, using the word 'thing' all the time to save the mind the effort of ferreting around for the right word.

'We have found', says Susan Williamson, 'that patients with severe language problems appear to go downhill faster than patients who exhibit only impaired memory.'

Some people will restrict their language to a few choice words that are used automatically. A British woman living in the Midlands says of her husband: 'I find I am having to put out clothes for him to wear, else he'll be wearing a summer shirt in the dead of winter, and if I remonstrate with him, then he says that it is perfectly alright and beautiful. His vocabulary is limited, and everything is "lovely" or "beautiful". His vocabulary is confined to the weather only, and when out he'll greet people, even if he does not know who they are, with "Nice bright day", but if unsuspecting friends carry on the conversation he puts on a face and says "Yes, you're right". The inborn gentleman in him rises to the top.'

In many cases, during the progression of the disease, it is as if a stranger emerges, entering the home with such stealth that other family members are unaware of the arrival until someone suddenly comments 'Dad just isn't like he used to be', or 'Whatever happened to the wife I knew?' For it can happen that there is a complete personality turnaround.

A Sydney psychiatrist says: 'The most predictable aspect of the disease is that the person will change — though having said that, and thinking about patients I have seen, even this is not so. Many delightful people remain delightful; many aggressive people, aggressive. It all depends on the individual and the areas of brain predominantly affected.'

Princess Yasmin says of her mother, Rita Hayworth: 'I have to steel myself each time I see her now. I'm her flesh and blood, but when I see her so helpless I almost have to disassociate myself, because she will say and do things that just pierce my heart.'

A London man recalls: 'June was irritable for about a year, and when she came to bed she would lie there mumbling. I thought she was simply talking in her sleep but I realised later that she was fully awake. There was a tremendous crash one night and I woke to find she was not in bed. She was in the lounge looking down at a lantern she had knocked over. She had tried to pull her dress on over her nightdress and it was all tangled around her neck and arms. I told her to come on back to bed, but she wouldn't come. At dawn I went out and found her in the back yard, sitting on the concrete with her back against the wall. It was the first time I was aware she had gone wandering like that, and it shocked me.'

For the dementing person, it is not he or she who is the stranger, but members of their own family. 'I can't leave my husband for a minute,' laments a Californian woman. 'He will walk out the door and get lost. He eats with his hands now, and often accuses me of being a stranger in his house. I can't cope much longer, but I feel terrible when I think of putting him away.'

Mrs Bobbie Glaze, a leading official with the Alzheimer's Disease and Related Disorders Association in Bloomington, Minnesota, said in 1982 of her Alzheimer-afflicted husband, a former civic leader and administrative vice-president of his company: 'He is now a statistic. He is permanently hospitalised, not knowing his family or speaking a word in the past four years ... It became frightening, living with this stranger who might push me or twist my arm or throw things at the television. The loving, gentle husband I once knew was no longer there.'

Everything that 'normal' people take for granted — looking at a clock and not only being able to see the time but also being able to *understand* the hour in relation to the day, or walking to the shops to buy a newspaper — is an effort for the dementing person.

When you ask a dementing person in the latter stages of the disease if he understands something you have just said, he will probably say that he does, when in fact this is an automatic response — the question hasn't really registered. More than likely by this time, he will have started to hallucinate, although hallucinations are not always an indication that someone has Alzheimer's disease. These 'city mirages' can sometimes be brought on by certain drugs or emerge from treatable conditions like delirium. It is when hallucinations follow a period of forgetfulness, vagueness, loss of everyday words, that there should be cause for concern.

A neighbour: 'Mrs Gore is always wandering down the road. Once, she was holding the heads of all the flowers she'd picked off in her garden and she accused me of climbing over the fence and taking them. I found her in my garden one day stealing my flowers. We all knew there was something wrong with her, but her husband was very embarrassed and never talked to anyone about it. What do you say to someone who comes into your garden and picks your flowers and doesn't know what she's doing? I was going to get on to her husband about it, but it wasn't his fault, poor man. What could he do to stop it happening again? You can't help talking about it when you see her wandering around like that.'

Although families are aware of their relatives' problems, they often have difficulty recalling exactly when the first changes emerged. Says Robert Butler of the Mount Sinai School of Medicine:

'The process is so insidious that colleagues, friends and relatives unconsciously begin to assume responsibilities that were once routine for the afflicted individual; a spouse learns to balance the chequebook, a secretary or a co-worker provides extra support to get the ailing individual through the work day. Even close acquaintances may dismiss bizarre behaviour changes — even as they begin to unconsciously avoid socialising with their friend. Often years go by before the peculiarities of behaviour and the declining intellect are viewed as symptoms of disease and diagnosed as senile dementia of the Alzheimer type.'

The disease takes its victims from the first stage, which includes forgetfulness, withdrawal, hallucination, suspicion, disorientation and confusion, into a mental darkness where everything is finally stripped from them. If kidneys, lungs or heart fail first, the sufferer, many doctors concede, is fortunate. And so are his relatives. Some people die within four or five years of being diagnosed. Others disintegrate slowly, watched by their despairing relatives. Australian singer and actress Jeannie Lewis says about her mother: 'Physically, she looks like something out of Belsen, but she eats still, which is strange. I don't think she knows who I am. She's been in bed for a year.'

The disease can go on, from beginning to end, for fifteen years or more. Maggie Millar, wife of the detective writer Ross MacDonald, said after the death of the man she had always called Ken:

'I did my grief three years ago. Ken hasn't really been here for a long time. I scattered him at sea. We'd talked about how we're all bio-degradable and how it would be nice to return to the earth. I get comfort from that when I walk the dog on the beach. I've had a flood of letters from around the world and telephone calls with questions about Alzheimer's disease. Most of the people who they say have it probably don't. I think it's like autism in children. No one's home. Their brain is tuned in on something only they know about. Just because we don't understand it, doesn't mean it isn't there. They tried to tell me Ken's brain was dead. I didn't believe it. Ken was peaceful, right to the end. Some Alzheimers are full of rage. One I know used to pummel his wife. At least I was spared that.'

The curtain rises on the last scene of this tragedy to reveal a character who has forgotten his lines. He cannot walk about his home, his stage, and he does not hear the reaction of the audience — in reality, the tears and despair of his family. He is stripped of the ability to recognise all that God gave him. In the worst case, left alone in his chair, he would not cry for help, for he does not know the word. He would starve to death, sitting in his urine and faeces. All manners and social customs have been eaten away. Despite the round-the-clock attention of his family, his dignity has eroded. He leans over to one side, mouth dropped open, saliva hanging down.

This is happening today in homes around the world, affecting the lives of rich and poor. The afflicted person wails. Hearing it in the night for the first time, a house guest might be alarmed, for there is something inhuman about it.

'The patient's light switch is still on, but there's no illumination,' is how one psychiatrist describes the final symptoms. Those who are still able to walk do so with a stoop, arms hanging down loosely, little steps, as if afraid they will tumble were they to take a longer stride.

'There is nothing left,' says a Berlin woman of her husband. 'He is just like a cushion padded out with foam. He sits in his chair and I sit in the other chair. Sometimes I watch television, and sometimes I just sit and watch him. He looks at his lap. It isn't any kind of life for either of us.'

When all faculties have gone, the sufferer becomes a dead weight. Lifting him from a chair or bed requires great strength. Sometimes the afflicted person will yell out as a relative tries to help him up. Perhaps he sees his helper as an ogre who wants to drag him to an evil place, for who knows what warped pictures that hallucinating brain is projecting.

The last stages are not a joyful prospect. For some, the condition may not be as severe as for others. The effects of the disease on the personality will vary, but one thing is certain. The afflicted person will not get better. Of all the challenges to medicine, the battle against Alzheimer's disease remains among the most awesome.

5

Finding out

For the third time in a week, your wife has gone out, forgetting to turn off the stove.

Your husband goes missing. He went to the shops one Saturday morning, and the police found him late in the afternoon, far away.

A brother doesn't go down to the local pub any more. His mates say he's so quiet nowadays. Doesn't seem to enjoy their company as he used to.

A friend's personality completely changes. Always kind and loving, she suddenly accuses you of stealing her teapot.

Such departures from 'normal' behaviour may be cause for concern. They could be warning signs that the relative or friend is in the early stages of Alzheimer's disease. Or they may be suffering from a temporary lapse of memory or be going through a period a depression.

How do you find out? How on earth can the doctors tell? They can't zip open the skull, have a quick look around for those telltale tangles and plaques, and make a diagnosis. Yet it is vital to find out if something other than Alzheimer's disease is to blame so that the condition can be treated. A large number of factors can bring on symptoms similar to the early stages of the disease, which makes diagnosis difficult. There might be some chemical imbalance in the blood, a nutritional deficiency in the brain, stress or depression, some type of toxic poisoning, a tumour or a virus. Any of these conditions could mimic the early stages of senile dementia, but unlike Alzheimer's disease they are treatable — and the earlier they are diagnosed, the better.

'Even for the specialist, positive diagnosis of a mild degree of mental impairment is not at all straightforward,' concedes Dr Amos Griffiths, of Oxford's Radcliffe Infirmary. Medical, neurological and psychological tests are made on a patient, not to search for tangible evidence of Alzheimer's disease, but to look for and eliminate other problems that might be mimicking symptoms of the disease.

Alzheimer's disease is such a feared condition among those who know of its devastation that the US Department of Health and Human Services, in a special guide prepared for health practitioners, says: 'Because the diagnosis of Alzheimer's disease carries with it such a dismal prognosis, you must display extraordinary care before pronouncing it. And because the only way it can be pronounced with absolute conviction is on autopsy, you must in effect back into a different diagnosis by discounting first all the other illnesses that might cause senile symptoms. Once you know what the diagnosis is *not*, you are left with just one probable explanation: Alzheimer's disease.'

Doctors who have confused patients referred to them are expected to consider a range of treatable causes. Factors that might have triggered the problem are:

Drugs Some 20 per cent of people with disturbed behaviour suffer from drug intoxication, researchers in a number of Western countries agree. This is hardly surprising when it is considered that 65 per cent of all prescribed drugs are for the elderly.

Dehydration In hot weather, old people can dehydrate within 24 hours. Drugs that help them to pass water add to the problem.

Depression and environmental changes Doctors and researchers have found that some people reach an acute state of confusion and depression following changes in their environment. Moves from one place to another can bring about a sense of loss.

Urine retention This is fairly common in elderly people and can bring about disturbances in the mind.

Constipation The two favourite topics of conversation among the elderly, it is said, are their financial affairs and their bowels. There is a great deal of truth in this, for the ageing begin to worry about security as the years pass. But bowel movement is of equal importance. Constipation makes them feel uncomfortable, they can develop incontinence because of the obstruction, and this can lead to the development of an acute confused state.

Pain It has been found that infection or pain causes severe confusion in the elderly. Sometimes the behaviour of a person is so disturbed that doctors do not associate it with a physical condition.

Tumours Doctors agree that there are a number of malignant lung tumours that cause severe confusion. It has been speculated that a fast-growing cancer extracts important nutrients from the system, which leads to disturbed behaviour or a delirious condition in some people.

About one in ten people over the age of 65 suffers from some functional illness, the most common being depression. This can bring on symptoms similar to the early stages of dementia; the sufferers speak more slowly, are forgetful, do not walk at their usual pace and avoid mixing with people. They are slow to grasp things when spoken to and give the impression of being dimwitted. In effect, they are victims of the stresses of life; researchers agree that depression is a collapse of the emotions and the physical makeup of the body. The condition can follow financial problems, the taking of too many drugs, marital difficulties, retirement, general ill-health, bereavement and the social decline and isolation that can accompany old age. Psychiatrists have established that those suffering from depression may exaggerate their distress; but an Alzheimer sufferer will have reserved emotions.

One of the first things the doctor considers, then, when someone has been showing signs of memory loss is whether the root of the problem is depression. The older the patient, the more prone he or she is to psychiatric illness. Dr Colin Godber, a British specialist in psychological conditions in the elderly, points out that to make a diagnosis in an older person showing the early signs of dementia an adequate history is needed — not just from the patient but from someone who knows him well. This is to establish just what sort of person he used to be and whether his present personality and behaviour match up with this. What sort of stresses and changes in lifestyle has he experienced in the past few years, months and weeks, and how do these tie in with any changes of behaviour?

One point doctors will watch for is whether families and friends will remember only the aspects of behaviour that have been a nuisance, such as sleep disturbance, general restlessness or aggression. But doctors also need to know whether the person has been unhappy, hasn't been eating much and has not shown much interest in life around him.

'The other problem in getting a history', says Dr Godber, 'is that the relative or neighbour questioned will often have decided what the trouble is, what its cause was and what solution should be applied. Thus, the onset of symptoms will often be dated wrongly from some event such as a bereavement, when in fact they were present, if less obvious, long before. This is frequently the case with dementia, where the patient's disability is covered up by a caring spouse, or with depression where exacerbation of a longstanding illness will be oversimplified as just a 'brief reaction' to a recent bereavement. In other cases, the patient may have become the scapegoat for a wider family problem. The descriptions of the patient getting more difficult may simply reflect changes in the family tolerance, rather than in his actual condition. This often makes it harder to monitor the responses to treatment, as a resentful family may be reluctant to recognise improvement or, by continuing to show their rejection, perpetuate the negative aspects of the patient's behaviour.'

In addition to getting down to the root of the problem through the family, doctors must also try to obtain information from the person himself. However, they may find they are up against a wall — the affected person may not cooperate, either deliberately or because he does not understand the questions asked. In the elderly, communication is often handicapped by deafness, blindness or a speech disorder not connected with the onset of any mental problem. Doctors find that depression is almost as difficult to diagnose as Alzheimer's disease. Some doctors find it easier to eliminate all other symptoms before looking at the question of depression or Alzheimer's disease. After all other tests have been carried out, and before leaping to a diagnosis of Alzheimer's disease, many GPs feel they owe their patients at least a trial of antidepressants and perhaps a session with a psychiatrist or psychologist if depression is the probable diagnosis.

While depression is frequently a red herring for Alzheimer's disease, American researchers agree that the most common cause of forgetfulness, confusion and disorientation in the aged — conditions that lead to depression or vice versa — is drug intoxication. The physiological changes of age often make the elderly more prone to adverse side effects and interaction between different types of drugs. Because they have a greater proportion of fat cells than when they were younger, the functions of their liver and kidneys have decreased. This means that drugs take longer to clear out of the system. In addition, some people have trouble taking their medicine properly either because they did not understand the doctor's instructions or because they forgot when they last took their pills. The first system that breaks down when the drug burden becomes too great is the nervous system. So when a patient is brought to a doctor for an evaluation of some mental problem, the first thing the GP might do is eliminate all drugs for a trial period. In many cases this successfully clears up the confusion and when essential drugs are reintroduced the person is able to manage on less.

Appendicitis, heart attack, even the flu or gastric trouble can throw the mind out, causing confusion, memory loss and disorientation in people who are advancing in years. These conditions rarely cause mental impairment in the young and middle aged, but they can be enough to disrupt the balance of a brain that has already started to undergo the normal changes of ageing. When the equilibrium is shifted by any external stress, even something like a head cold, the brain is often the first internal part of the body to show signs of the strain. Doctors used to dealing with mental conditions are careful not to jump to conclusions. When someone is brought to them with all the appearances of dementia, experienced physicians will still suspect almost anything as being the cause, particularly if the symptoms have appeared suddenly, rather than over a period of several months. The US Health and Human Services Department advises doctors:

'The odds are that you will not find a treatable cause for the symptoms — only an estimated 15 to 30 per cent of cases of senile dementia can be reversed — but you must look anyway. The consequences of mistaking a potentially treatable disorder for irreversible Alzheimer's disease are too devastating to allow for anything but a no-holds-barred approach in the workup of a patient with senile symptoms.'

Doctors experienced with dementia cases know some of the immediate things to watch out for. For example, confusion brought about by some toxic effect on the brain usually brings about restlessness, and the person often needs constant attention; dementia sufferers are usually, but not always, quiet. However, the symptoms might overlap, and that can confuse the doctor.

Dr Godber says his experience as Consultant Psychogeriatrician at Southampton's Moorgreen Hospital has shown that allowance always has to be made for difficulties in communication or cooperation when assessing answers given by a patient. Doctors have to take great care, he says, to keep questions as simple and brief as possible, and they have to avoid embarrassing the patient with questions that only point out his shortcomings.

'Many old people get labelled as confused — or worse still as senile or demented — simply because they are uncooperative or apathetic or simply because they are expressing bizarre ideas,' he says.

Doctors have drawn up various tests to help them make an early evaluation. One doctor working in Australia uses a series of tests based on muscle reflexes, and this is described later. Dr Godber, however, asks a few simple questions: the day, the date, the patient's age, the name of the prime minister, some events in the patient's own life in recent days. If the person gives the day and the date correctly, he need go no further; confusion is ruled out. In patients in their eighties or nineties, an error in the month or year would not matter too much if they got their age and one of the other questions right.

Should the patient turn out to be not confused, a consultant will start to look for a 'functional' illness such as depression or a state of paranoia, or some sort of emotional disturbance, and will also look for a hearing or speech disorder. Dr Godber believes that if someone is confused, the history will indicate whether it has been a 'chronic deterioration', suggesting dementia, or a more recent development which may be associated with an illness, a change in environment or the use of medication.

Often, to pull out the real answers, many hours have to be spent with a confused person because examinations can include everything from a scrupulous physical examination to a comprehensive round of electronic and photographic procedures. Because of the cost of some equipment used in making a diagnosis, tests are often carried out in one major medical centre and can take a whole day.

Before any electronic tests are made, specialists will run through a list of 'diagnostic pointers'. A typical list used by Dr Godber always includes questions about the patient's history and mental state. When looking for depressive illness, he will try to establish whether there has been pessimism; suicidal thoughts; loss of appetite, weight, sleep and interest; depressive ideas of guilt, persecution and a belief the person is ill; anxiety; loss of confidence; fear of being alone or going out; demand of attention; hysterical behaviour; aggression; grumbling and moaning; crying; moodiness; apathy; self-neglect; loss of pride; poor recovery from physical illness; bereavement; change of home; restlessness; wandering, often at night; paranoid ideas. Having received answers to these historical questions in the search for mental illness, Dr Godber will next turn to the mental state of the person and try to establish his present mood; whether he is depressed, whether life is 'not worth living' and whether his memory, particularly his recent memory, is good but concentration is poor. If most of these factors are present, it is likely the person is suffering from a depressive illness.

When testing for dementia, Dr Godber looks for the following symptoms, in their usual order of appearance: progressive impairment of memory, with recent events most affected; loss of day-to-day household and intellectual skills; self-neglect and risk of accidents with gas taps and similar household appliances; wandering, especially in active people, as disorientation worsens; variable loss of ability to mix socially; inability to dress; incontinence of urine, often beginning at night; incontinence of faeces; difficulty in walking and feeding. Moving on to the present mental state, the psychogeriatrician looks for an impaired recall of recent events by asking a person his age and so on. But the consultant will also test the person's recall of longer standing events by asking such questions as his date of birth.

In trying to establish alternative causes for Alzheimer symptoms, doctors might carry out physical examinations: taking blood counts; testing the liver and kidney functions; looking at the calcium, phosphorus, sodium, chloride, potassium, carbon dioxide, sugar, vitamin B_{12} in the body; and carrying out chest X-rays. They may also arrange for a CAT scan, a PETT scan or an EEG test. Daunting though such names sound, the processes are painless and can help the experts make an assessment.

A CAT is a computerised axial tomogram — a complex X-ray machine that gives technicians a picture of the brain, unlike an ordinary X-ray camera which really only shows up the bones. Today's machinery is a sophisticated brother to the equipment first developed in the early 1970s by G.N. Housefield, an electronics engineer who introduced his EMI brain-scanning device in a London hospital and which was to win him and his colleagues the 1979 Nobel Prize for their research in physiology. The technique used today is basically the same. A metal 'hat', similar in appearance to a huge hair drier, is placed over the head, and thousands of X-ray beams pass through the skull towards sensing devices which send electronic signals to a computer. The computer puts together an image of part of the brain, which then appears on a TV screen. It may show evidence of multi-infarct dementia, clots of blood putting pressure on the brain, tumours and the obstructed movement of the cerebrospinal fluid in the brain. Most importantly, it will possibly show changes associated with Alzheimer's disease, such as a shrinkage in brain tissue, areas of decay and enlarged ventricles. But the tangles and plaques cannot be picked up; they need to be located through a microscope, which is, of course, not possible through the skull.

A PETT scan — positron emmission transaxial tomography — is based on the work of an American team, Louis Sokoloff and his colleagues at the National Institute of Mental Health Laboratory of Cerebral Metabolism at the University of Pennsylvania. It allows medical investigators to study the physical functions of the living brain without the use of surgery. Sokoloff and his fellow scientists recognised that because glucose is the main source of brain energy, the less glucose used by parts of the brain, the less active those regions are. Alzheimer-diseased brains, it has been found, use less glucose than healthy brains. The PETT scan enables researchers to monitor how the brain is using glucose when they 'read' a picture on a TV screen. With this system, investigators are able to see what activity is going on in the brain when a person is talking, thinking and sleeping. They can observe what happens in the brain when drugs are taken, and they can see when disease begins to disrupt its normal functions. One encouraging finding for the elderly is that their brains continue to work on well, at least to the age of 83. With the aid of the PETT scan, scientists looked at data on the brain activity of 21 people between the ages of 18 and 83. The researchers reported that there were no statistically significant reductions in the amount of glucose used in many brain regions of the older people. The conclusion is that despite minor changes in memory which occur with ageing, normal adults can expect to maintain a high level of brain function throughout their lives.

An EEG test involves the use of a piece of equipment known as an electroencephalograph. In a painless exercise, wires are attached to the head with a special paste and these record the electrical activity of the brain. If the activity of the brain waves is slow, it suggests abnormality.

Some specialists might arrange for a lumbar puncture, also known as a spinal tap. It involves inserting a needle into the spinal column in the region between the pelvis and the ribs and drawing fluid from the spine. If it sounds ominous, it is not painful after a local anaesthetic has been administered, although there might be some later discomfort. The purpose of this operation is to draw off a small amount of cerebrospinal fluid, which circulates between the spinal cord and brain. Any malignancies or infections responsible for memory loss can be detected when the fluid is analysed.

Any of these physical or electronic examinations may indicate the reasons for a person's confused behaviour. If the tests suggest dementia, the next stage is to establish just how severe it is. Specialists need some basis on which to work, and having recorded the person's present condition, a consultant will arrange to see him again, probably in six months. If the degree of dementia has not worsened significantly, the likelihood is that the person does not have Alzheimer's disease. Just how confused the person is at the outset can be assessed by special questions. These may be along the lines of the simple test used by Britain's Dr Godber: day, date, age. Guidelines laid down for American specialists suggest ten simple questions: Where are we now? Where is this place located? What is today's date? and such like. A score of nine to ten means the patient is not confused; six to eight, slightly confused; three to five, moderately confused; 0 to two, severely confused.

Such simple tests are not always adequate to locate mild forms of dementia, and some specialists include other questions. They may ask the person to remember a list of three or more items and then ask in five minutes or so what the items were. Other patients are asked to count backwards, to interpret proverbs or to explain cartoons. Sometimes a person will be asked to copy a simple diagram shown to him. The accuracy of the copy helps a doctor to assess the degree of confusion.

Although all these tests are far from conclusive, they help to build up a picture. Relatives and friends are also asked personal questions about the person. Has he had any 'accidents' with his bladder or bowel? Can he move without help from bed to chair? Can he move about on foot or by wheelchair without assistance? Is he able to take care of his hair and teeth and use the toilet independently? What about dressing — can he accomplish that without help? Can he bathe without assistance? Can he cope with chores around the house? Is he able to travel alone by public transport?

Those who are severely impaired will not be able to do any of these things, whereas those with moderate impairment will be able to manage dressing and washing. People who can care for themselves and travel alone on trains or buses probably have no impairment, or very little.

There is a further test that can help doctors to make up their minds whether a person has Alzheimer's disease. Very simple, but very telling, it is known as the Face-Hand Test. The specialist sits opposite the person, who has been asked to close his eyes and place his hands on his knees. The doctor then strokes the patient's cheek and the back of one hand. The patient is asked to say which cheek and which hand are being stroked as the doctor moves from cheek to cheek, hand to hand. It has been found that even when the test is repeated with the person's eyes open, 80 per cent of those who performed poorly with their eyes closed do no better.

Another clue that could point to Alzheimer's disease is in the way a person walks. In many victims of the disease, the posture is stooped, the gait slow and the arm swing virtually absent. They may take mincing steps from a flexed stance with the feet well apart — the *marche à petits pas* is how it's sometimes referred to. The hands might be cupped. And there are some reflexes that appear with Alzheimer's disease which are not present in healthy adults. When the area around the chin and mouth is tapped, the person's lips pucker. Those afflicted with the disease also tend to grasp whatever is placed against their palm, and when pressure is placed against the sole of the foot, the toes turn downwards.

British neurologist J.M.S. Pearce usually gets a good first impression. The suspected dementia victim looks vacant, lost and bewildered. He often claims he is not ill and does not know why he has been brought to a doctor. There is frequently a history of forgetting names and faces, a tendency to lose familiar possessions, and errors of judgement at his place of work or in behaviour. The personality is bleached, and interests have waned. The neurologist says depression often occurs at an early stage — sometimes before loss of intelligence is shown. In his experience, the features of established cases include an impairment of memory, deterioration of intellect, a change in personality and behaviour, and emotional disorders. Certain basic reflexes — sucking and pouting, grasping, a contraction of a muscle in the chin when the palm of the hand is scratched — are usually present in the early stages of Alzheimer's disease and are a good indication of an organic problem. However, these signs cannot be read to distinguish atrophy of the brain from something like a tumour or multi-infarct dementia. Absent in an Alzheimer case are any signs of paralysis on one side of the body, spasticity — lack of muscular control because of brain damage — or any loss of the senses. There may be evidence, however, of some speech disorder and indications of inability to manipulate objects. Dementia associated with an inability to coordinate the face, tongue and lips and an inability to express and comprehend, indicates Alzheimer's disease, providing there are no accompanying headaches, vomiting or epilepsy.

Dr Pearce supports CAT scanning: 'a non-traumatic and painless test which has greatly simplified investigation.' It can exclude tumours and give a measurable index of the size of the brain and the ventricles. EEG readings, though, he says, seldom aid the diagnosis. A British colleague, Dr Griffiths of the Radcliffe Infirmary, does not exclude the EEG. Standard investigations, he says, may reveal an underlying organic disease responsible for a confused condition. It may also be valuable to exclude dementia in cases where a confused state has been ruled out because it is then likely that pseudodementia is present.

Across the Atlantic, Dr Marshal Folstein of Johns Hopkins University Medical School, Baltimore, has been impressed by the fact that EEG readings appear 'diffusely slow' in patients who have the classic symptoms of Alzheimer's disease. But he concedes it is 'extremely difficult, if not impossible' to achieve early diagnosis through procedures presently being used.

'Clinical symptoms that identify Alzheimer's disease really take several years to develop to the point that permits confident diagnosis,' says Dr Folstein, who has also devised a series of tests of memory, language skills and other functions for Alzheimer suspects. He insists that follow-up checks and clinical examinations are required to detect the sequence of symptoms and to rule out other neurological disorders. Specialists also need to be on the lookout for acute cases of confusion and depression. Although a person suffering from such conditions can cause great hardship and anxiety for their families, these problems can be treated with reasonable success. As Dr Godber says: 'This applies just as much when the conditions are superimposed on a dementing illness, where they are still eminently treatable, often with great relief to patient and family alike.'

In rare cases, a brain biopsy may be carried out. This involves giving the person a general anaesthetic, cutting into a small portion of the skull and removing a tiny sample of brain tissue from a so-called 'silent area' of the brain — away from areas related to speech, for instance. The problem is that it is the speech areas that are most likely to be affected early and would show the changes that are being sought. This means that a biopsy may miss a badly affected area and show relative normality when significant disease is in fact present.

Although biopsies can sometimes help with an assessment, surgeons are generally reluctant to put someone through the trauma of a major operation so he can be tagged as a 'confirmed' Alzheimer victim. There are usually enough clues in behaviour and other tests to help doctors make an assessment of the type of dementia. The experts won't always get it right first time every time. But as the months progress, the person's behaviour will either confirm their original assessment or provide them with more clues for making an accurate diagnosis the second time around. If a biopsy has not been carried out, the only way to be 100 per cent certain about Alzheimer's disease is to cut open the brain after death and examine tissue under the microscope.

Words such as 'diagnosis', 'biopsy', 'CAT scan', 'tumour' or 'brain disease' are frightening for many non-medical people. They are cold, clinical, belonging to another world, another dimension, to some future time, way beyond George Orwell's 1984. Perhaps words like 'dementia' and 'depression' conjure up visions of asylums from the Dark Ages. They certainly didn't belong in your home when the doctor first mentioned them to you. You couldn't associate them with the once-vibrant, intelligent person you spent so many years with.

The words aren't used to frighten you or your family member or friend. They are simply used by medical experts to identify certain conditions or identify instruments used to assess those conditions. Just what effect they have on you as an individual depends on the picture your own brain paints for you. For some, medical terms are terrifying; for others, they are no more frightening than 'table' or 'book'. Just as our brains work differently, producing various thought processes, so changes in the brain, if and when they come, will vary from one person to the next.

A loss of memory does not necessarily mean Alzheimer's disease. But it should be watched, and if it continues, it should be referred to a doctor.

6

Possible causes and research

What causes dementia of the Alzheimer type? Should we stop eating out of aluminium pots, live in the country away from car and factory fumes, eat home-grown vegetables that haven't been sprayed with pesticides, remove ourselves from everyday tensions, avoid bumps on the head, stop taking medicines, drink less alcohol, get more sleep?

We could try each and every one of these and still fall victim to the devastating disease. On the other hand, something in that list, some change of habit, might save us. Right now, there isn't a researcher in the world who can say with 100 per cent conviction 'I know what brings it on.' The Nobel Prize awaits the scientist who finds a cure.

What is known about the disease is that it affects between 5 and 10 per cent of all people over the age of 65. Among those who have been diagnosed as having progressive dementia, Alzheimer's disease accounts for between 50 and 60 per cent. It has been said that a look at patients and residents in hospitals and nursing homes suggests that Alzheimer's disease strikes more women than men, particularly those of a lower social status. But health workers explain that women tend to live longer than their husbands, who might have cared for them at home until their deaths. The social status belief is also unfounded — wealthy families tend not to send their relatives to nursing homes, because they can afford the luxury of a live-in private nurse. Alzheimer's disease is not selective.

It can strike in the forties and fifties, affecting people from all walks of life across a broad spectrum of intelligence. You can live in a caravan or in a mansion; spend a life of leisure or slog away from dawn till dusk; you can live in the snow or reside in the sun, in the desert or beside the sea, on a mountain or in a valley. In the Soviet Union, the Ministry of Health has set up health spas in the Black Sea region where rest, diet control, weight loss and a pleasant environment are all part of an attempt to prolong life by ten years or more. Nevertheless, Soviet people get Alzheimer's disease, just like anyone else. Whoever you are, whatever you do, no matter what you eat, whatever the colour of your skin, you are in the Alzheimer lottery.

Although great progress has been made in the past ten years in developing instruments and research tools, uncovering the cause of the world's fourth biggest natural killer is still beyond the scope of today's scientists. One neurologist comments: 'It's like peeling off the layers of an onion — the more we peel, the more there are.' And Dr Gene Cowan, Director of the National Institute of Mental Health in Washington, concedes: 'We could be decades away from finding the cause. Even then, we would only be talking of prevention, not cure.'

Researchers agree that diet might have something to do with it. But the benefits of certain foods might be less effective with some people than with others. Stress could be a contributing factor. But then, people who are able to cope with stress better than others might still become demented because of some other factor.

Herbert Weiner, an American authority on psychosomatic diseases — bodily illnesses caused by mental factors — says: 'We need to account for the fact that only some predisposed persons fall ill; others seemingly have a greater adaptive capacity and therefore remain in good health. Events and experience have an impact on the minds of persons. Some adapt to experience, others do not. If they do not and disease ensues, we may ask how the received experience is translated into physiological changes and bodily events.

How does psychological distress that may signal adaptive failure become transmitted into disease?'

He suggests that the psychosomatic idea is based on the theory that social and psychological factors play a role in the predisposition, inception and maintenance of many diseases.

Some researchers agree that disease can follow bereavement or some change in a person's life with which he is unable to cope. He feels helpless and induces a state of hopelessness throughout his entire body. Another school of thought suggests, like Herbert Weiner, that people are 'predisposed' to illness. They might carry a tinderbox of genetic or biochemical factors that needs only a spark — stress, a secondary illness, a shock — to ignite it. But as one authority, Franz Alexander, at the Chicago Institute for Psychoanalysis, suggests, 'being predisposed to a disease doesn't mean one will get it.' Psychological maturity, a general state of good health and pleasant surroundings may prevent it.

Ideas can be tossed around, theories expounded, but nobody can be totally sure about the cause of Alzheimer's disease. Instead of distress passing into the body to cause disease in, say, the heart, does it remain locked in the brains of some people, manifesting itself in the tangles and plaques? It's possible, say the scientists, but they add that they don't really know.

But there is hope. Years of examinations and research have produced a great many clues and some positive findings. They may not all add up to one definitive cause, and some of the leads go full circle and take researchers right back to where they started, but they all help in the process of elimination.

Obvious questions facing today's researchers are whether the disease has viral, biochemical, hereditary or environmental origin. The answers lie deep within the human brain. Animals don't get it naturally, although scientists say they can produce neurofibrillary tangles in rabbits, a development discussed later in this chapter. It seems the disease is something we as humans bring upon ourselves, or are exclusively prone to.

Just what is it that causes our brains to go haywire, while every other creature on earth is spared the disease? Is it a problem of the New Age, or has it been with us since the beginning of human life? That it was isolated as recently as 1906 leaves us wondering for how many centuries, how many thousands of years, plaques and tangles have been forming in the human brain, unrecognised because the technical ability to see them had not been developed.

If a simple theory can be put forward, it has been suggested that what you don't use, you lose. Researcher Dr Warner Schaie of Seattle says: 'The use-it-or-lose-it principle applies not only to the maintenance of muscular flexibility, but to the maintenance of a high level of intellectual performance as well.' And Nancy Denney, consulting psychologist at the Institute on Ageing at the University of Wisconsin, comments: 'What one does during one's life makes all the difference.'

Some researchers hold the belief that staying socially involved might help to keep dementia at bay, for it has been found that mental deterioration is most rapid in old people who withdraw from life. It is important, say researchers, to remain mentally active and have a 'flexible' personality. One study has found that those able to tolerate ambiguity and enjoy new experiences in middle age retain their mental alertness best through old age. The idea, it is suggested, is to remain physically and mentally active right through one's life. When a halt is brought to thinking or working, it can speed up the end. Research in France, for example, showed that within three years of compulsory retirement, 37 out of 100 bricklayers died.

Until early adulthood, the human brain is still growing: very quickly at first and then at a slower rate so that by the age of twenty it has created something like 10 billion non-reproductive nerve cells. Having reached its peak production, the brain begins to age, losing some 50 000 neurons every day. They simply die away, never to be replaced; and although this rate may seem alarming, it is normal. Another change takes place: ageing brings about the destruction of dendrites, the branchlike extensions through which the main body of the cell receives messages from cells in other parts of the body.

Scientists at the Albert Einstein College of Medicine in New York, using a special machine to count the cells in various parts of the brain, have found that with Alzheimer patients there is a much greater loss of large neurons in the cerebral cortex — the grey, wrinkled outer cover of the brain associated with thought and memory — than in a cortex that has aged normally.

Does our immune system get a false reading on our brain cells, believe they are harmful invaders, and set about destroying them? The fibres at the core of neuritic plaques are composed of an abnormal protein. These may be, just may be, signs of a defect in the body's immune system. Normally the system attacks and destroys bacteria, but sometimes, possibly as a result of ageing, the immune system may turn against the body's own tissue. If that tissue consists of brain cells, the immune system may manufacture antibodies and launch scavenger cells on 'seek-and-destroy' missions against brain neurons.

There have been some steps foward in the study of the chemical make-up of the brain and its role in Alzheimer's disease. The nerve cells secrete a substance called acetylcholine, an important chemical transmitter, one of about 25 chemicals that help send messages from one nerve cell to another. In manufacturing acetylcholine, the brain uses an enzyme called choline acetyltransferase — choline, for short. This enzyme fades away in the brains of the elderly and can be decreased by as much as 90 per cent in the brains of those with Alzheimer's disease. In simple terms, with little choline there is little acetylcholine, and when there's not much of that there's poor communication between the nerve cells. The result, researchers conclude, is the destruction of memory, learning and judgement.

Until recently, it was thought that the loss of acetylcholine in the cerebral cortex and in the hippocampus — the memory bank — was due to the death of neurons originating in these areas. However, American scientists have found that destruction of nerve cells in the cerebral cortex does not result in the loss of acetylcholine. This is an important discovery, for it told Dr Joseph T. Coyle and his colleagues at the Johns Hopkins University School of Medicine that the cell bodies that produced acetylcholine in the cortex were located in some other part of the brain. They searched ... and found. The location of these neurons was deep within the base of the brain, in an area known as the nucleus basalis. How did they find this out? They injected a chemical toxin into the nucleus basalis area of rats and, as expected, found this destroyed the nerve cells in this area. The effect was a dramatic loss of the important acetylcholine in the cerebral cortex. What happens in the brains of rats also happens in the brains of humans. So the onset of Alzheimer's disease could lie deep within our 'control centre', the nucleus basalis.

When the scientists caused this imbalance in the chemical makeup of a rat brain, they produced a change similar to that brought about by Alzheimer's disease. Realising the importance of the discovery, Dr Coyle teamed up with a colleague, Dr Donald Price, to look further into the role of the nucleus basalis region in Alzheimer's disease. Their first post-mortem was carried out on the brain of a 74-year-old man who had succumbed to the disease. They were excited by their findings: the loss of neurons in the base of the brain was an astonishing 90 per cent greater than the loss in a normal brain of corresponding age. What's more, some of the surviving cells in the nucleus basalis showed those telltale neurofibrillary tangles. The scientific detective work continued. Five more post-mortems were carried out, this time on patients in their late fifties or early sixties who had died in the final stages of dementia. The studies showed the same nerve cell destruction in the nucleus basalis area.

Taking their research further, Coyle and Price concluded that the other pathological (disease-causing) feature of Alzheimer's disease — neuritic plaques in the cerebral cortex — was the result of the destruction of neurons from the nucleus basalis. This changed earlier thinking that the death of neurons originating in the cortex was the root of the problem. Important though the findings were, they left Dr Coyle commenting: 'We need to know a lot more about what the nucleus basalis does and how its projections to the cerebral cortex are organised.'

What is known is that the nucleus basalis is in a position to accept and send messages between other parts of the brain, including the areas affected by Alzheimer's disease. The study by Coyle and Price and their colleagues has identified for the first time a specific population of nerve cells that could be the culprits behind Alzheimer's disease. Now scientists wonder whether dying acetylcholine-producing cells trigger the formation of plaques. There seems little doubt, however, that the loss of choline, a key factor in the production of vital acetylcholine, is characteristic of Alzheimer patients.

New drugs are continually being tested today at hospitals, medical centres and universities, and victims of Alzheimer's disease are using them with either their own or their relatives' consent. There are brain stimulators, general rejuvenators and some remarkable potions that promise to turn on the fountain of youth. As a cure for Alzheimer's disease, however, drugs have so far been unable to help. Comments one geriatrician: 'So far, we haven't been able to prevent it, reverse it, or slow it down. Success would undoubtedly be worthy of a Nobel Prize, and the commercial rewards would be enormous.'

Ian Stout and David Jolley at Manchester's Withington Hospital say a tantalising hope presents itself: that chemical engineering designed to bypass lost enzyme systems or prevent the breakdown of precious neurotransmitters might reverse some elements of this, the most common dementing illness. Such breakthroughs have yet to be achieved — satisfactory substitutes for acetylcholine and choline have not been produced.

Researchers hold the belief that increasing the amount of this transmitting substance, or preventing its excessive breakdown, or prolonging its action when it is working between two nerve cells, might help the neurons that have not been destroyed by the disease. Experiments with drugs have been made with healthy human volunteers and laboratory animals, and they have been found to enhance memory. Just to make sure that the 'positive' drugs are working in the right area, researchers have used what are known as anti-cholinergic drugs on volunteers and these have temporarily produced a loss of memory similar to that seen in Alzheimer sufferers. The 'positive' drugs consisted of choline — that substance used by the body in the manufacture of acetylcholine — and lecithin, the dietary source of choline, which is found in all membranes.

The brain draws a great deal of its supply of choline from the bloodstream. What we eat generally determines the level of choline in the blood. Protein foods such as fish, beans, egg yolks and meat have a high choline content. Interestingly, when lecithin is given to 'test' patients, it increases the level of choline in the blood more than an injection of choline itself.

Researchers have tried adding choline and lecithin to diets in a number of clinical trials with Alzheimer's disease patients, but Dr Suzanne Corkin of the Massachusetts Institute of Technology reported after the first experiment: 'Test results in general are not promising.' She thought, though, that many of the studies were inconclusive because of a disorganised experimental system. She then tried further tests under stricter conditions, using eighteen patients with Alzheimer's disease with conditions ranging from mild to severe. They were each fed a preparation of lecithin for a period of eighteen weeks. But there was no significant improvement in memory. Says Dr Corkin: 'Even isolated improvements in memory test scores or in home performance did not raise the mildest Alzheimer's patient to the level of a healthy elderly subject.'

Again, the researchers suggested that an erratic test performance and a large variation in the test scores could have masked the effects of minor improvements. Does Dr Corkin believe that feeding lecithin over a long period can slow the progression of the disease? The only answer, she concedes, is yet more studies.

At the Duke University Medical Centre, in Durham, North Carolina, several avenues of research have taken place, including a trial of lecithin treatment. Eighteen patients, aged between 50 and

69 with mild to moderate dementia, received either lecithin or placebo — a 'dummy' drug — over a period of 24 weeks. At the start of the study and at the end of each eight-week session, the people were tested for mental status. The results were again disappointing.

Dr Albert Heyman, who supervised the tests, says: 'One of the major observations in this study was the decline in cognitive function (awareness) that occurred during the 24-week period of the trial. Greater disorientation, further disturbance of immediate memory, and an increase in the severity of aphasia [speech disorder due to brain impairment] during this comparatively short period of time were indicated by the cognitive test results.' Rapid deterioration, says Dr Heyman, is a serious obstacle in evaluating possible therapeutic agents in Alzheimer's disease.

Researchers still believe that many of their answers lie in that important transmission substance, acetylcholine. Perhaps, it was suggested a short time ago, something could be done about reducing the rate at which the body breaks down acetylcholine. Tests showed that a drug called physostigmine reduces the rate, and it was decided to administer it to ten patients with Alzheimer's disease. The study, conducted by Dr Kenneth L. Davis and Dr Richard C. Mohs at the Mount Sinai School of Medicine in the City University of New York and at the Bronx Veterans Administration Medical Center, produced positive results. Memories improved. The patients, ranging from 50 to 68 years of age, were carefully selected — particular care was taken to test those who were certain of having Alzheimer's disease and not multi-infarct dementia — and they were given varying doses of drug or placebo. The patients responded better to a recognition memory test when receiving physostigmine than when receiving the placebo, which consisted of nothing more than an ordinary salt solution. So researchers had some indication that retarding the acetylcholine breakdown in the brain could at least partially reverse memory problems. They say partially, because physostigmine did not improve the patients' performance in all the awareness tests. It had to be administered, too, in varying doses from subject to subject for best results. Not only that, the drug's effects lasted only 30 minutes or so, and long-term use can have an adverse effect on the heart and lungs. In addition, the drug is injected, which is not considered practical in treating elderly demented people.

How would it help if physostigmine was used along with lecithin? Dr Bruce Peters and Dr Harvey Levin, at the University of Texas Medical Center, tried combining the two, injecting physostigmine just under the skin and feeding lecithin to Alzheimer patients, and the doctors noted an improvement in memory. But they had to be careful with the amount of physostigmine administered. 'Too little isn't effective and too much can actually worsen memory functions,' says Dr Peters.

There seems to be no doubt, though, from the trials at the Mount Sinai School of Medicine and at the University of Texas Medical Center, that lecithin provides additional choline for acetylcholine while physostigmine prevents its excessive breakdown. Dr Peters, however, issues a caution:

'Although the physostigmine–lecithin treatment definitely augments memory in certain Alzheimer's disease patients, we do not wish to make any claim beyond that. We have no reason to think that this has any effect whatsoever on halting or modifying in any way the cause or natural consequences of Alzheimer's disease.'

Why such reserve after an apparently encouraging study? In his work, Dr Peters has found that best results with the physostigmine–lecithin treatment are obtained in patients with mild or moderate dementia. Those who have moderately severe or severe symptoms are not really helped. And even some patients who initially showed improvement in memory stopped responding to therapy — some after 18 months, some as early as a year after treatment began. Of his test patients, he says: 'We believe that all of them will cease to respond eventually. This medication should be viewed as assisting a function, but the function is progressively worsening despite the effects of the medication. At some point, the medication ceases to overcome the progression.'

Like technicians looking for the cause of a breakdown in a massive telephone junction box, medical researchers work on, probing neurons, examining the transmitting substance, testing the brain's sensitive receivers. Scientists continue to produce drugs, and tests show they help memory, but that's as far as the research goes. Nothing yet beats the inevitable progress of Alzheimer's disease. As Dr Herbert Weingartner of the National Institute of Mental Health in Bethesda, Maryland, commented after a series of memory-enhancing tests with a new drug, DDAVP: 'It's important for people to appreciate the fact that we're not yet near achieving a promising therapeutic leverage on Alzheimer's disease.'

At America's National Institute on Ageing Laboratory of Neurosciences, researchers have been exploring another approach. Instead of trying to stimulate the neurons which produce acetylcholine, or trying to slow down the degeneration of the transmission system, scientific investigators have been looking at the function of the acetylcholine 'receiver'. It is possible that by stimulating these receptors by some outside agent they could take over where nature has left off?

Once again, they used laboratory rats to try out their theories. They injected the animals with a drug called oxotremarine and found that it stimulated areas that, in a human brain, are associated with memory. In Alzheimer victims, although other brain cells degenerate, the receptors remain relatively unaffected. Researchers think, therefore, that despite the loss of the transmitters, the receivers can still be stimulated and some functions of the brain can continue.

Alan Davison of the Institute of Neurology at the National Hospital, London, believes there may be a chemical abnormality in the brains of people with Alzheimer's disease. The fact that some people retain a high intellectual capacity with no alteration in perception throughout their lives suggests that where severe impairment occurs, it may be associated with some disease process. He is in accord with his American counterparts that acetylcholine is less active in people with Alzheimer's disease, and this has a direct relationship to the degree of disease damage and mental status. However, he says that not all people show the same changes in their brain transmitters.

The belief that brain transmitter deficiency is responsible for deterioration in mental functions is also held by European scientists. Dr Marco Ermini of the Institute of Experimental Gerontology at the University of Basel, Switzerland, supports this concept and suggests the answer to the problem may lie in drugs. 'The symptoms of senile dementia may be alleviated by the administration of drugs which normalise neuronal metabolism and neurotransmitter function,' he says.

Among drugs claiming to bring brain cell chemistry back to normal and help the transmitter system work is hydergine, in use for more than ten years, and which Dr Ermini describes as 'outstanding'. It has multiple effects on the transmitter system of the brain, but one of its main functions appears to be restoring interplay between transmitters. It also reduces blood pressure. Just what the benefits of hydergine are can be seen from the results of a study conducted by another Swiss specialist, Dr S. Koberle of the Geriatric Hospitals, Basel. She has tested the medical and psychological effects of the drug on elderly retired people who were given hydergine over a three-year period. Dr Koberle used 148 volunteers, whose average age was 63, but none had any physical or mental disorder. For three years, half the group were given hydergine, the other half an ineffective placebo.

In the group on hydergine, it was found that symptoms of tiredness, dizziness and emotional unstableness decreased. The conditions increased among the group being given the 'false' drug. The effects on the IQ were also interesting. At the start of the trial there was no significant intellectual difference between the groups, but after three years those on hydergine had improved. In verbal tests, performance in the first year in both groups increased; then it fell off in the placebo group, whereas it was maintained in the hydergine group. Hydergine, Dr Koberle says, can be tolerated in long-term dosages with no side effects and few significant changes in blood pressure. But it wasn't just the effects of hydergine that fascinated Dr Koberle. Most people, irrespective of the group they had been in, reported at the end of the trial that they felt better. 'An increase in the feeling of well-being appears to reflect the increased attention given to trial subjects,' she says. The effects of care and attention given to dementia sufferers is examined later.

A doctor who has been using hydergine for more than ten years, Ronald McConnachie of the Chesterfield Royal Hospital, Derbyshire, has found that memories do improve through use of the drug. Although the majority of British doctors are still sceptical about the effects of drug therapy on the failing brain, Dr McConnachie says: 'In my experience, from clinical trials and from research, I believe there is now sufficient evidence to accept that hydergine does have a small but definite effect on the symptoms caused by the failing brain.'

His beliefs are strengthened by the medical reports he has studied from around the world. More than 1300 people with mild to moderate brain failure have been tested with hydergine and all tests have shown that the drug assists thought processes, behaviour, emotional stability and everyday living capability. Side effects, he says, have been remarkably few — occasionally there has been an increase in restlessness and confusion.

Another Swiss doctor who has had considerable experience with hydergine emphasises that a biochemical approach to treating dementia is just one way of tackling the problem. Dr Dieter Loew believes other forms of treatment should include improving the nutrition and the social environment of the elderly, as well as correcting any deficiencies they may have with hearing, seeing and feeling, for example. A person with true dementia is likely to benefit from drug treatment, he says, but patient selection is very important: in mild forms of dementia it is difficult to see any effect of the drug, and in advanced cases the disease tends to resist the treatment.

Leading neurologist Dr Robert Katzman, of New York, is also hesitant in handing out too much praise to the effects of drugs. Referring to hydergine and related drugs, he says they could improve performance in some individuals, but they 'are not miracle drugs.' He told the annual meeting of America's Alzheimer's Disease and Related Disorders Association in 1983:

'We're still a long way from preventing or curing the disease. We don't know enough about the disease yet to achieve a breakthrough. In the meantime, it's very difficult, but I think we all have to remain sceptical. We have to remain very cautious when we see media claims of any kind of dramatic breakthrough in treatment of Alzheimer's disease. We know it's a terrible disease. We are all hopeful there will be a breakthrough someday soon, but we can't expect it to come overnight. Rather, I think we can expect that gradually some drugs will be introduced that will help memory, certainly in the early part of the disease. Gradually, more potent drugs will be found, and finally, scientific research will give us some real hint as to what causes the disease, and then we can do something very important about it. You will have to bear with us. It's going to be a few years yet.'

Almost monthly, some group of researchers somewhere announces an achievement. Often, the progress is parallel to other advances, but in the overall battle to find a true cause and cure, Alzheimer's disease continues to emerge the victor. But there are always glimmers of hope.

In April 1983, a New York University Medical Center team announced a breakthrough with the drug naloxone, used mainly in addiction treatment. Their tests show there was at least a temporary improvement in the condition of patients treated. 'Previously it was all gloom and doom,' Dr Eugene Roberts, one of America's leading researchers who led the team, said when the findings were announced. 'Now there is an open window with a ray of sunshine bursting through.'

The new studies showed that naloxone relieves memory loss and improves cognitive functions in many areas of the brain that can be tested. The theory is that naloxone blocks the damaging effects of the disease on the brain cells by counteracting the damage caused by the body's own natural substance, encephalin. It was Dr Roberts who in 1950 identified a substance known as gaba, a key chemical believed to be involved in the progress of Alzheimer's disease. Since then it has been found that gaba is central in epilepsy, Huntington's disease and schizophrenia. Dr Roberts, explaining the working of the drug, says: 'It appears naloxone helps to increase circulation in the brain by blocking these encephalins and allowing the various neurons necessary for any intelligent function to do their job.'

A few months after Dr Roberts made his announcement, the Illinois State Psychiatric Institute revealed that it was testing a promising new memory pill. Tests with animals using the drug CI-911 have shown that it can help to restore memory, Dr Lawrence Lazarus said. 'The question now is whether it will work in patients with Alzheimer's disease.'

Dr Lazarus, director of the institute's geriatric psychiatric programme, says several drugs were tested, including lecithin and choline for possible memory-restoring abilities, but the results had not been encouraging. How could they test the memories of animals? Dr Lazarus explains that mice were given mild electric shocks to induce a state of amnesia. Creatures given the drug were quicker to recall how to run through mazes than those that did not receive it. Dr Lazarus's researchers also administered the drug to elderly rats and noticed that brain waves, believed to be associated with memory, improved. Tests on humans, which were to continue until the end of 1984, were being conducted like other drug-testing systems: patients are given either the drug or a placebo. In the early stages of the tests, patients and their families reported dramatic changes in memory. 'They want to keep taking the drug after the study is over,' says Dr Lazarus, 'but that's not possible. It might be a placebo effect or it might be the drug. We are cautiously hopeful.'

Like Switzerland's Dr Koberle, Dr Lazarus is well aware that some people feel better after being given 'something', even if it is a neutral agent. This 'placebo effect' is brought on by the patient's high hopes, the desire to please the researchers, the stimulation of being a subject in an experiment, and body changes brought on by the person's postive mood. Because of the placebo factor, repeated trials of new drugs are always necessary, as well as checks on patients for months or years afterwards. As the US Department of Health and Human Services says: 'This is where many drug "bonanzas" fail the test.'

There is no doubt among scientists that somewhere in the chemistry of the brain they will find a solution to the problem. Just why Alzheimer brains burn less glucose and whether this is important is also being studied. Doctors have known about this slower process since the end of the 1940s as machines to read the mechanism of the brain improved. Today's PETT scan system gives doctors a clear picture of the functions of the brain, and they are able to see how slow the glucose-burning process is.

Most of the oxygen used by the brain is spent burning the glucose. When the activity of a particular part of the brain increases, the rate at which it burns glucose increases. And because most of the glucose and oxygen are supplied by the blood, the local blood flow goes up. Changes in glucose and oxygen use and in the blood flow are used by scientists to determine the areas of the brain involved in activities such as hearing and speaking. Researchers believe that the decrease in glucose and oxygen use in the brains of Alzheimer patients are effects of the disease rather than the cause.

'Several lines of evidence suggest that the decrease in brain metabolism — chemistry — are important,' says Dr John Blass, of New York's Burke Rehabilitation Center. 'Conditions which reduce the ability of the brain to burn glucose, for instance, decreases in the levels of oxygen or glucose in the blood, characteristically impair brain function. Judgement and mental acuity are among the first functions to change as oxygen is lowered; for instance, as one ascends in an unpressurised airplane. Severe and prolonged reductions in the supply of oxygen and glucose to the brain kill nerve cells and nerve cells die in Alzheimer's disease. Cells which make the chemical acetylcholine are exquisitely vulnerable to changes in the supply of oxygen and glucose to the brain, and such cholinergic cells are characteristically damaged in Alzheimer's disease.'

Dr Blass points to studies in England and America that suggest that in an Alzheimer brain there is damage to the chemical machinery which burns glucose. The studies suggest that not only is the 'thermostat' set differently, but the 'furnace' is also damaged. These considerations suggest that the decreases in brain metabolism may contribute to the brain damage in Alzheimer's disease.

'The interest of researchers in this area has waxed and waned over the years and appears to be increasing again. That brain sugar metabolism is altered in Alzheimer's disease is well established. Even if these changes simply reflect the sickness and death of brain cells in this disease, they may still prove practically useful as biological markers of the presence and progression of the disease.

'If the impairments prove to contribute to the sickness and death of brain cells, they would be yet more important. The more we understand about why and how brain cells are damaged in Alzheimer's disease, the more hope there is of coming onto better ways to ameliorate the process.'

A suggestion that has raised great controversy among researchers is that aluminium may play a part in the development of Alzheimer's disease. Post-mortems on the brains of those who died from the disease have, in some cases, shown a suspiciously large amount of the metal in cells that also contain neurofibrillary tangles. Some scientists came to the conclusion that if aluminium was found among the tangles, could they not induce tangles by introducing aluminium to a normal brain? Obviously they had only laboratory animals to work on, but their theories were proved correct. Injecting aluminium salts into animals produced tangles.

Such early studies — they were made in 1965 — inspired Canadian researchers to look further into the role of aluminium. In 1976 they announced their findings: there was an increase of 10 to 30 times the normal concentrations of aluminium in the brains of people who had died from Alzheimer's disease or dementia of a similar type. Which came first, though: the aluminium or the disease? Did aluminium deposits cause Alzheimer's disease by acting as a toxin, or did the metal accumulate as a result of changes brought on by the disease? A flurry of experiments began. These tended to show that the presence of aluminium in the Alzheimer brain was indicative of a deteriorating system, but the answer to the 'chicken or the egg' question could not be positively defined. Aluminium is found in the brains of the healthy elderly, but to a much lesser extent. Recent studies have helped to reveal the role of aluminium in Alzheimer-type dementia and normal ageing by pinpointing the site of aluminium concentrations in the memory bank of the brain, the hippocampus. With the aid of a new and extremely sensitive method of identifying and analysing the make-up of biological tissues in Alzheimer's disease, scientists have found that 90 per cent of the brain's nerve cells with neurofibrillary tangles had aluminium in the central part of the cells. Yet nearby cells that did not have tangles were virtually free of detectable amounts of the metal.

One researcher who supports the belief that aluminium plays a significant role in the cause of Alzheimer's disease is Dr Leopold Liss of the Ohio State University School of Medicine, Columbus. He believes it can be absorbed and controlled with the use of sodium fluoride, which would bring it together in the intestines and then be excreted instead of being absorbed by the body. Dr Liss wanted to satisfy himself that aluminium did produce neurofibrillary tangles, so he added it to the diet of rabbits. The tangles formed. He now knew for certain what he had to fight against. Because all humans are exposed to aluminium from the environment through food, dust and water, Dr Liss came to the conclusion that the body contains a protective barrier against the metal. In some individuals, he theorised, this barrier is faulty, allowing aluminium to enter the brain and cause degeneration of the neurons.

The doctor points out that the underlying chemical principle for preventing the absorption of aluminium has been used for years in veterinary medicine to fight fluoridosis in cattle. For this, an aluminium substance is administered to combine with fluoride and prevent its absorption into the body from the intestines.

Dr Liss's treatment reverses the technique by administering sodium fluoride to prevent absorption of aluminium. He has been encouraged by the lower level of aluminium found in the body fluids of people in the early stages of Alzheimer's disease who have been treated with sodium flouride. 'We are trying to help individuals who can still communicate with us, who still have sufficient attention span and can follow certain commands and participate in a number of tests,' Dr Liss says. He administers the treatment three times a day at mealtimes, and in some instances it has shown encouraging signs. But in other cases, progressive degeneration towards complete dementia has continued.

Whenever a theory is expounded, there is often a scientist or a group of researchers who will find a reason to knock it down. Some researchers have suggested that aluminium gains access to the brain through the blood stream. Following studies on animals at the Michigan State University, a substance known as parathyroid hormone has been blamed for producing increased absorption of aluminium from the intestines and increased amounts of aluminium in the brain's grey matter.

However, researchers at the National Institute of Mental Health Adult Psychiatry Branch at St Elizabeth's Hospital, Washington, DC, have found no evidence to link an aluminium increase in Alzheimer brains with a general overload of the metal in the body's fluids. Researchers David Shore and Richard Wyatt compared aluminium concentrations in the blood of people with Alzheimer's-type dementia against that of other, healthy, people of all ages and found no significant difference. Neither could any significant difference be found in a comparison of the aluminium in 'brain fluid' taken from the spine. The scientific investigators also looked into the amount of parathyroid hormone in the blood of patients with Alzheimer's dementia as well as in patients of the same age and sex without the disease. That they found no great difference between Alzheimer patients and healthy people led them to speculate that the hormone might not be a factor in the development of the disease.

Whatever it is that allows aluminium into the brain, researchers at the University of Toronto have been working on ways of removing it. They have been experimenting with a drug called deferoxamine, and first results have been encouraging, although one of the problems has been overcoming what could be debilitating and dangerous side effects. The Canadian attempt to remove aluminium from the body follows the same track as Dr Liss — using a chemical or drug to bind the aluminium together so that it can be flushed from the system.

To lessen our chances of 'getting it', should we keep away from aluminium? Throw out our cooking pots, remove the tin shed at the bottom of the garden, stop taking antacids (a source of aluminium), swap all our aluminium picture frames for wooden ones?

Obviously, most of these measures would be extreme and unnecessary. However, some scepticism may be forgiven about the use of aluminium cookware, especially as some neurologists advise relatives of Alzheimer sufferers — those with a greater risk of getting the disease — not to use uncoated aluminium pots. Other experts say there are no grounds for such advice. And Dr Liss hopes the metal will not be found to be the cause of Alzheimer's disease. As he says, there is no way of avoiding it; it's in the air, in our water, in the ground.

Could a virus be the culprit ... a slow-acting virus that comes alive in the brain after lying dormant for years? If tests on chimpanzees are anything to go on, a 'time scale' transmittable virus could be responsible.

In the late 1960s, researcher D. Carleton Gajdusek reported that degenerative brain disease in chimpanzees had been produced by injecting their brains with brain tissue from people suffering from Kuru. Kuru is a central nervous system disorder unique to certain native tribes of Papua New Guinea. It produces a rapidly progressing dementia leading to death, as does Creutzfeldt-Jakob disease. Both diseases are caused by viruses. Gajdusek's findings — the transmission of Kuru and Creutzfeldt-Jakob disease — have been replicated, and it was this that gained him the Nobel Prize. Alzheimer's disease has not been found to be transmittable among humans, but there have been case reports strongly suggestive of accidental transmission of Creutzfeldt-Jakob disease by corneal transplant, from an affected donor, and by neurosurgical operation, presumably via contaminated instruments. Kuru was transmitted in New Guinea mostly by the eating of human brains. Gajdusek found it to occur mostly in first-born sons and their mothers; this was explained by the custom of feeding the brains of opponents killed in battle to these family members.

The slow virus theory is far from dead. A possible breakthrough has now been reported from the University of California in San Francisco. Dr Stanley B. Prusiner says he and his team believe they have found the stimulus of Alzheimer's disease, and if they can verify this 'it will have enormous consequences'. Dr Prusiner and his researchers have been studying forms of albumen — a protein solution — called prions. These tiny bodies are so small that a single one cannot be detected under the powerful electronic microscope; when hundreds of these submicroscopic infectious particles group together, they are still as minute as a polio virus. The germ, which is neither a bacteria nor a virus and apparently contains no genes, is known in full as a proteinaceous infectious particle. If it is eventually proven to have no genes, it will be the first organism discovered without them. It is unique in another way: the Californian researchers, who have come close to isolating the germ after nine years' work, say its self-propagation seems to violate the basic laws of biology.

The prion's unusual make-up, the scientists believe, possibly explains why some diseases fail to stimulate responses from the body's defence system. Could the organism, they wonder, be so bizarre that the body may simply be unaware of its presence? Dr Prusiner says he has no idea how the prion survives and multiplies without genes, which control reproduction in all other forms of life. 'Once we have isolated the prions,' says the researcher, 'we can work out their structure and reproduction. I don't think that will prove a major problem. In turn, this could lead to great medical breakthroughs, although these could be some years off.'

Are these prions responsible for Alzheimer's disease, lying dormant in the brain for perhaps twenty years before setting to work on the neurons? The answer is unknown, but Dr Prusiner is able to study them because they tend to lump together into a size big enough to be detected under the microscope. His investigations are based on finding out how someone acquires a prion — whether, for example, it forms from an infection and how long it takes from the moment of a possible infection to the outbreak of the sickness.

At Sydney's Macquarie University, molecular virologist Dr Millar Whalley believes that the prions might contain a small amount of hidden genetic information. He points out that Crutzfeldt-Jakob disease could have an incubation period of up to 50 years. The implication of this is that the seeds of dementia are sown in childhood. If this could be proved, scientists generally believe, a vaccine might at some stage be developed which could prevent dementia and even go so far as preventing the ageing process in the brain. But these are only possibilities. The research continues.

Further work is being done on the fibres that make up the neurofibrillary tangles. These fibres are also abnormal proteins, and some researchers are of the opinion that because genes control the manufacture of proteins the abnormalities could reflect the working of a defective gene. Genes are inherited. Does it mean that Alzheimer's disease can be passed on through families? The indications are that it can.

7

A family fate?

Jim sits in the kitchen sipping tea, snatching a few moments to himself. Shirley, 56, is in the lounge in front of the television, but her eyes are on the floor. A supervisor, Jim has had a sour experience at work this day: 'Jim', said his boss, 'I know you need all the time you can get to be at home, but I just can't be responsible for your wife.'

Jim could see all kinds of problems looming up from that warning, and if anybody doesn't need more worry it's him. His wife has Alzheimer's disease, and if it wasn't enough to see her losing her memory, he has also shared the sorrow of *four* other members of Shirley's family succumbing to similar symptoms at a relatively young age. 'I can't say for sure whether they all had it,' says Jim, who lives in an inner Sydney suburb. 'They died when doctors weren't really looking for Alzheimer's disease in people. But the indications are that it's been running in Shirley's family. You can be sure that my married daughter, who's 29, is concerned about it.'

Tragedy no. 1 was Shirley's mother. She passed away in 1954 at the age of 58. She had become vague, lost her memory, could not speak and was unsteady on her feet. One day she went into a coma and was rushed to hospital, where she died. A post-mortem revealed a tumour, but in discussions with doctors since then Jim learned that the tumour could have come up after Alzheimer's disease, or a similar disorder, had set in. 'Alzheimer's disease wasn't being looked for then, so it was the simplest thing to say that the tumour had caused all the problems,' says Jim.

Tragedy no. 2 was Shirley's oldest brother, Jack. He had become vague and was prone to wandering away from the house. He was also plagued by heart trouble. One day in 1963 he wandered on to the highway, was struck by a car, and killed. He was just 50 years old.

Tragedy no. 3 was Shirley's elder sister, Helen. When she was only 49, Jim realised there was something wrong with her. She started to lose her memory and was becoming very vague. She was still driving her car, though, and one day she had an accident — ran into somebody. She couldn't go to court; she wasn't aware of what she had done and she had to be represented. After a while, a glazed look came to her eyes and she lost the ability to speak and walk. When she couldn't feed herself or look after herself, the family put her into a nursing home, where she passed away. Doctors said cholesterol, blocking her arteries, was the principal cause of death.

Tragedy no. 4 was Shirley's younger brother, David. He dropped dead in 1974 at the age of 42. 'His death was due to cholesterol, but I have this terrible feeling that if he'd lived on, he would have developed Alzheimer's disease. After all, if cholesterol runs in the family, as it seems to because Shirley has it as well, and all the family members have also had declining mental faculties, it seems to me that David would have fallen victim to this brain disease, too, if he had lived.'

Tragedy no. 5 was Shirley herself. In 1978 Jim noticed a slight change in her personality. She tended to leave the stove on and kept asking what day it was. In the end, Jim bought an electric clock which showed the day, date and time, and for a while Shirley was able to read it. When her memory got worse, the doctor told Jim that somehow the cholesterol in her body was much to blame. Shirley was referred to the Royal North Shore Hospital, Sydney, where a neurologist operated a CAT scan on her. There was no real evidence of mental impairment, the specialist said, but by a process of elimination he and his colleagues concluded that Shirley had Alzheimer's disease. Since that diagnosis, in 1980, Shirley's condition has steadily deteriorated. 'She still recognises faces, but she doesn't know who they are,' says Jim. 'She doesn't know her sons or daughter by name, and I have to help her with all her toilet affairs. She still manages to feed herself if I cut the food up small for her, but she gets it everywhere.'

Each morning Jim drops Shirley at his daughter-in-law's home or leaves her with one of his two sisters and then goes on to work. He picks her up late in the afternoon, brings her home and cooks for her. He knows the future holds little promise. He's concerned about getting enough time off to be with Shirley, and he's worried that his boss is one day going to say: 'It's your job or your wife.'

Anyway, convinced that Shirley's decline will continue, Jim knows that the day will come when he won't be able to handle her. 'I've already been to look at one nursing home. It was so bleak — nothing like home. But I know that Shirley will end up there or somewhere similar. There comes a point when it all becomes too much for the family.

'I've told my daughter she mustn't worry. She's another generation and there's nothing to suggest there's anything wrong with her. Of course, I understand her concern. When it comes down to it, all we can really do is hope and pray.'

'Am I likely to get it?' This is one of the most common questions asked of doctors by the children of Alzheimer sufferers. The answer is that they have a greater than average chance. Two or three people in 100 aged 65 or older will fall victim, but the odds increase four times or more if a close relative is affected.

'There's a simple way of understanding the risks involved,' says a British neurologist. 'Imagine a large casino containing 200 people, 100 of them relatives of Alzheimer victims, the rest having no known history of the disease in their family. The "clear" group stand equally spaced around a roulette wheel which has been divided into 100 sections. Two of those sections are marked with a star. When the wheel stops spinning, the stars will stop opposite two of the players — your next victims of the disease. At another table, eight stars have been marked off, and when the wheel stops it will identify eight out of the 100 "players" who will be struck.'

The first significant study of family links was noted in 1925 when a German researcher, F. Meggendorfer, carried out post-mortems on 60 people with senile dementia. Sixteen of these had had dementia problems in their families.

In a 1952 Swedish study, investigators examined eighteen patients who were found after post-mortem examination to have definitely had Alzheimer's disease, the term of illness having ranged from three to thirteen years. Three cases of family links were found: a father and his child, and two mothers and their children.

With interest growing among Swedish scientists, another study was conducted in the early 1960s. Of 217 patients who had lived in the two biggest mental hospitals in Stockholm, evidence of senile dementia was found in 29 family members — twenty sons or daughters and nine parents. Making allowances for people who could not be interviewed, it was concluded that the risk of getting the disease was about 10 per cent for sons and daughters and nearly 21 per cent for parents. In other words, this study shows that a parent who sees a son or daughter get the disease has about a one in five chance of falling victim.

That the son or daughter of a sufferer develops the illness may not have anything to do with genes. It may be the family environment which is to blame. However, studies so far indicate that the closer the relationship, the higher the risk.

It presents a big family worry. One woman in her early fifties rang her cousin, whose mother had the disease, and told him: 'Every time I can't remember a name, every time I can't recall where I put something, I say to myself "Is this it?"'

'They tell me Alzheimer's disease isn't catching,' says a Melbourne woman. 'But I'm beginning to wonder. My mother got it and now my husband has it. Perhaps living in close proximity to someone who has it sparks it off. Whatever the reasons, I couldn't cope with two sufferers on my hands. My mother is now in a home. I had no option. I'll be really worried if I start forgetting things.'

Dr Steven Matsuyama, Research Geneticist at the Veterans Administration Medical Center in Brentwood, California, and Dr Lissy Jarvik, Chief of the Psychogeriatrics Laboratory at the Center, have brought together the results of studies by eight research groups — six in Europe and two in the United States. After a careful analysis of the studies, the two Americans concluded there was a higher family incidence of Alzheimer's disease, but no clear cause could be attached to genes. The eight research groups had conducted eleven family studies over a period from 1925 to 1981, and eight of the studies showed that there was a risk of parents getting the disease; the risks ranged between 1.4 per cent to 33.5 per cent. Eight of the studies also found risks ranging from 2.2 per cent to 19.5 per cent existed for the children of a parent who had Alzheimer's disease.

Dr Matsuyama and Dr Jarvik combined data from three studies made in 1952, 1963 and 1978 to work out the combined risks for children. Based on 1146 children of 265 dementia sufferers, the researchers found there was a 7.5 per cent risk up to the age of 80 years. This was three times the general population risk of 2.5 per cent. The findings meant that more than seven people in 100 faced the chance of becoming demented if one of their parents was a victim. By the age of 85, the combined risk had risen to 11 per cent, still three times the general population risk. Beyond the age of 85, the risk seems to increase even more, say Dr Matsuyama and Dr Jarvik, but study details are not adequate for an accurate analysis. (It should be emphasised that the risk of developing dementia for *anyone* is of the order of 1 to 2 per cent for all ages, 10 per cent for those over the age of 65, and 20 per cent for those aged over 80.)

The Americans say there is an erroneous assumption that because a genetic condition is inherited it is unmodifiable and incurable. 'Clearly, such is not the case. A good example is the prevention of mental retardation in the genetically determined disorder in phenylalanine metabolism [a body acid associated with adrenaline]. Hopefully, concerted research efforts in dementia of the Alzheimer type will soon be followed by empirically based treatments and methods of prevention equally successful for relatives at risk.'

There is no clear-cut pattern of inheritance from the limited number of studies made on genetic factors in Alzheimer's disease, which leads some researchers to think that several genes are involved which interact with environmental factors. Scientists have noted that Alzheimer sufferers often have abnormal chromosomes — the thread-like structures that house genes in body cells. These chromosomes pass on genetic information from one generation to the next. Normally, there are 23 pairs of chromosomes in human cells. But in Alzheimer's disease sufferers, a higher than usual percentage of body cells contain too many or too few chromosomes. And among those chromosomes, some defective ones have been found. Like two evil twins, Alzheimer's disease has been linked with Down's syndrome — mongolism — the birth disorder in which there is an extra chromosome. Down's syndrome sometimes shows up in the same family, and people with this condition also frequently develop Alzheimer's disease. In fact, the affected cells in an Alzheimer brain closely resemble those found in an older Down's syndrome brain. Some researchers are convinced that the brain changes and clinical symptoms of Alzheimer's disease occur in all Down's syndrome patients who live to the age of 30 or more. There is speculation, too, that Alzheimer's disease is linked to the advanced age of the mother at the time of the victim's birth.

Some of our chromosomes contain genes that govern the production of certain proteins, and these proteins are found in increased
amounts in the blood of Alzheimer victims. What has interested
researchers is the discovery that a particular gene often occurs in
association with a particular disease. This helps investigators to 'read'
the type of disease someone may be susceptible to; they simply look
for specific proteins produced by these genes. But this doesn't work
all the time.

In trying to understand incurable disease, medical researchers can
only go on 'tendencies'. They can only present their findings to the
world, give an opinion, and allow people to come to their own
conclusions. Some of the evidence, though, is very convincing: like
the incredible story of two neurologists who turned medical detec-
tives to trace Alzheimer's disease back through the generations to
one of two members of the same family who died at an early age in
a tiny town in southern Italy in 1790. The result of their investigations is that many of the family members who are living in the
United States and Europe today, people in their twenties and thir-
ties, are very worried. For their family history shows a record of
pre-senile dementia.

Long before CAT scans were invented to give scientists pictures
of the human brain, a young neurologist at Yale University was
asked in 1962 to examine a 35-year-old man who was often depressed because of his erratic memory. Dr Robert G. Feldman believed the man's troubles were more than emotional, and after various tests diagnosed the trouble as premature senility. He found
out that his patient had relatives in the Calabria region, and these
had died at an early age. He wrote to officials in the town of Nicastro and obtained municipal records on the deaths. In 1963, Feldman
published a report on family links in Alzheimer's disease. But he
didn't stop there. He tracked down other afflicted relatives in the
American states of Florida, California, Pennsylvania, West Virginia
and Connecticut. He also asked healthy family members to allow
him to do fingerprint studies, analyse their chromosomes and take
blood counts. What he was hoping for was a clue, a common denominator, that would enable him to predict and, dare he hope, halt
the onset of pre-senile dementia in the family volunteers. Unfortunately he could find no biological markers, and he was not helped
by the limited technology of the late 1960s.

Unknown to Feldman, across the Atlantic the scene was being set for astonishing developments in the American researcher's work. In 1972 a French neurologist, Dr Jean-Francois Foncin, was consulted about a supposed brain tumour in a 44-year-old woman. She had been earlier diagnosed as schizophrenic, and she was now becoming increasingly agitated and unable to care for her nine children. Because the CAT scan was still being developed, Foncin carried out a PEG test — pneumoencephalogram — in which air is injected into the sac surrounding the spine. Foncin could find no evidence of a tumour. But he was intrigued to find enlarged ventricles in the brain of such a young person. A brain biopsy was performed, and from an examination of the minute piece of tissue that was removed through a small hole in the skull, Foncin was able to see the telltale plaques and tangles of Alzheimer's disease.

Believing strongly that in cases when people so young are inflicted, the family history as well as the patient should be examined, Foncin set out on what was to be a fascinating example of medical detective work. First, he interviewed the woman's husband and found out that her father had died at an early age in a nursing home in Calabria. This turned out not to be a nursing home but a state mental hospital. Foncin wrote to the hospital asking for more details about his woman patient's father. The answer did not surprise him; the man had died of dementia after some years as a patient. Foncin could not let his investigations stop there. He made more inquiries in France and learned of other family members who were affected by mental problems. What was needed, he decided, was a thorough investigation. He obtained a grant from a private foundation and set off for the small town where the family originated — Nicastro.

The Frenchman did a thorough job. He obtained copies of photographs of the dead family members, photographs that are traditionally enclosed in the base of the coffin along with the name and dates of their life span. Among the dead, he found the name of the father of the young woman he had examined in Paris.

Next, he went through all the records at the local cathedral and the town hall and built up a list of family members who had died before the age of 50. He was interested to learn that many of the relatives who died young in two particular families had not died in Nicastro but in another town — where the old state mental hospital was located. Unable to find any more information to help him, he

returned to Paris, where he gathered together all published literature on early-age family cases of Alzheimer's disease. Among the
reports was the work of the American, Robert Feldman. The town
wasn't mentioned, but a reference to municipal records led Foncin
to guess that it was Nicastro.

He wrote to Feldman and thus found out why he had lost track
of so many patients in recent generations: they were in America,
under the care of Feldman. Foncin, who was now director of the
neuropathology laboratory at La Salpetriere Hospital, Paris, and
Feldman, chief of neurology at University Hospital and the Boston
Veterans' Administration Hospital, agreed to get together to compare notes. Foncin arrived in Boston with a computer printout
identifying 1200 relatives of the 35-year-old man Feldman first examined back in 1962. The family members were not all blood relatives, and the two neurologists were unable to work out which of
the two original family members was the transmitter because both
had died at an early age. But their findings did reveal that among
the 35 family members identified as having had the disease, the
symptoms started in their mid-thirties. There were positive changes
in behaviour by their early forties, and death followed by the age of
48 or 49 in all cases on both sides of the Atlantic.

Cases of pre-senile dementia were suspected of being connected
with families in the past, but because of family embarrassment or
the lack of records, its occurrence had, according to Dr Feldman,
been considered sporadic. 'When a young person was afflicted,' he
says, 'the condition was often concealed. Even now, people think
that dementia at 70 or later is normal. It's not normal. It's a disease.'

Foncin, acknowledging that hereditary indications can be worrying for those who are now young and healthy, says: 'Mercifully,
in Italy the family didn't know about genetics. Most family members were labourers or manual workers. They said this was over
their heads. When a family member became affected, the afflicted
one was protected and cared for as a child.'

The family members now living in Europe and America and who
are aware of the links have told researchers they are willing to
cooperate in the hope of perhaps tracking down a common factor. Some of the family group say they are hesitant about marry-
ing or having children because of the dementia background. Dr
Foncin has worked out that in the family tree he has compiled,
if one parent is affected with the premature form of dementia,

there is a 50 per cent chance of offspring developing the illness at an early age.

Alarming as these findings are for one family, they are not conclusive proof that Alzheimer's disease is hereditary for everyone else. There are hundreds of thousands of other cases who have no history — at least, no known history — of Alzheimer's disease, and there are hundreds of thousands of sons and daughters and grandsons and granddaughters who didn't get it even though an elderly relative did. Researchers agree, though, that there is an increased risk among families, and if the findings of Feldman and Foncin are to be considered, environmental factors cannot be seen as a cause. Lifestyles in Calabria are of course different from those in Paris, as the environment of Paris is different from that of West Virginia or Pennsylvania.

In 1980, the United States Department of Health and Human Services commented in a paper prepared for health practitioners: '... one's genetic legacy would be an important factor, but by no means the only factor in determining whether one will develop Alzheimer's disease.'

Since then, Foncin and Feldman have disclosed their findings, and although they alone are not enough to form conclusions, they add more pieces to the puzzle. Every time a new study into possible genetic links is made, the case for a hereditary factor becomes more credible.

Researcher Leonard Heston, from the University of Minnesota — his papers were among those studied by Matsuyama and Jarvik to work out their risk figures — came up with some worrying findings in a study of 30 people with Alzheimer's disease. Compared with the general population, he found a higher frequency of Down's syndrome and blood disorders such as Hodgkin's disease and leukaemia among family members. He speculated that a genetic defect is causing problems among the cells affected by Alzheimer's disease. He concluded that the earlier the onset of dementia, the more severe the course of the disease; and the more severe the disease, the greater the frequency in family members.

There is the consideration, too, that families who believe they are free from any recent history of mental illness might have ancestors who developed the same tangles and plaques that remained undetected throughout the development of medical science until they were isolated in 1906 by Alois Alzheimer.

Researchers believe that genetic research may provide the key to accurate diagnosis, and the search continues for specific biological 'markers' or indications; if a person has a certain gene, scientists would like to be able to say for sure that a disease will develop. Chromosomes, those structures that house genes, are attracting most attention from scientists. They have found that with advancing age, more cells appear to lose their chromosomal material, particularly in women. In people with Alzheimer's disease, this chromosome loss appears to be greater than in normal elderly people. However, the general feeling among Alzheimer specialists is that the chromosome loss is not enough to go on as a guide to those who are at risk of developing the disease. They point out that even if changes in chromosomes are detected, this could be brought about by any number of environmental factors.

At the Veterans Administration Medical Center in Brentwood, California, researchers have been looking at another genetic marker through what is known as philothermal response. In these tests, they base their research on the knowledge that cells have a tendency to migrate towards warmer temperatures. Preliminary findings reveal that cells from patients clinically diagnosed as having Alzheimer's disease respond abnormally to a warmer temperature, possibly because of a defect in the cells. After tests with a special temperature gauge, known as a microslide, were carried out, researchers Steven Matsuyama and Lissy Jarvik reported:

'Whatever the reason, when cells from patients with dementia of the Alzheimer type are placed at the cooler end of a microslide, far fewer of them reach the warmer end of the microslide after a few hours compared to cells from persons of similar age who do not have dementia of the Alzheimer type. Perhaps their cells are slower or disoriented — as are the patients themselves. There may be many reasons — they remain to be examined. Even before the precise biologic mechanism ... is uncovered, however, the philothermal response may become a useful diagnostic test for dementia of the Alzheimer type.'

Question from a member of the public to a panel of dementia specialists at a meeting of the Alzheimer's Disease and Related Disorders Society in Sydney: 'Is Alzheimer's disease hereditary? My mother is in her late eighties, in a nursing home in excellent physical health, but confused and forgetful. At 51, I now notice my memory is not good for remembering events and incidents. Physically, I too am excellent. Can I help myself? When I look back on my mother's life, I realise how very clever she was in covering it up.'

Answer: 'Alzheimer's disease does run in some families — and can start at any age — but this is rare. If your family has a number of members with the disease — providing diagnosis is accurate — then your risk is increased ... If you are concerned about yourself, you should see your doctor. Most cases of Alzheimer's disease come out of the blue, and the rest of the family is unaffected. There are many conditions other than dementia which lead to memory difficulties.'

As Dr Peter Davies of New York's Albert Einstein College of Medicine comments: 'The genetics of Alzheimer's disease is an area which is still very difficult to investigate. A significant problem in this area of inquiry is that a confirmed diagnosis is impossible without either biopsy or autopsy, procedures that are not very common.'

However, he and other specialists believe that further investigation of the genetic aspects of Down's syndrome and Alzheimer's disease may provide a new route to identifying the cause of Alzheimer's disease.

8

Another viewpoint

In an old-fashioned surgery in a Melbourne suburb, an elderly doctor sat waiting for his patients. They had been dropping away for months and now hardly anyone came. If anyone needed a doctor, someone said, it was the doctor himself. He was in his seventies, and advanced medical techniques had passed him by. He was a little slow on the uptake, and sometimes the chemists recommended a better type of medicine than he prescribed.

As his patients fell away, the doctor become lonely and boredom crept in. The bottle became his closest friend. Finally, sympathetic colleagues pulled him away from the practice and found him a single room in a teaching hospital, where he became a talking point. They put him under CAT scan equipment and, they concluded, the poor fellow had simply become 'old and mad'. They couldn't do a thing for him. It was necessary to find him somewhere to live, and the best thing, they all agreed, was that he should be certified and placed in a state mental health institution. But there were no beds available.

The case of the doctor who became a helpless patient came to the notice of a young Dutch psychogeriatrician who believed there was no such person as a hopeless case, at least not until he had been allowed to treat the patient. Dr Cees van Tiggelen took his elderly colleague into his care. The result was that less than five months after giving up the medical practice and going to the teaching hospital the elderly man was back home with his wife and declaring that he was going to enjoy the rest of his life. He had improved so much that when a conference of general practitioners was called to discuss 'Assessment of Psychogeriatric Patients', he took an active part, demonstrating that 'old and mad' is not always irreversible.

In a block of flats, a 73-year-old retired fitter, a widower for fourteen years, tried to look after himself with the help of his children, home helps and the meals-on-wheels service. One day, during her daily phone call to him, his daughter noticed how confused he was. He started talking about people looking at him and said there was a hole in a picture on the wall through which someone was constantly watching him. His daughter took him to a doctor who, unable to find anything obviously wrong, said the problem must be due to his age.

The next night, at 3 am, he rushed from his flat with a hammer and began smashing it on the concrete floor of the corridor, yelling and screaming at those he said were persecuting him. Two frightened elderly neighbours called the police and his relatives, and he was taken to hospital. He was diagnosed as being acutely psychotic. After further examination, doctors put the problem down to one of senility and he was discharged, his relatives being told to ensure he took six different tablets each day. For the next eighteen months, the man went on a merry-go-round of expensive private hospitals and nursing homes. At one stage he wandered off on to a busy street and nearly walked under a tram. He was sent to a mental health institution.

Yet by February 1979, a few months after his admission to the institution, the man was living independently in a flat again, looking after himself and, apart from one injection a month, taking no medication. He had a few memory problems, but his condition had improved immensely.

Both the elderly doctor and the man with delusions of persecution had received treatment with vitamin B_{12}, administered by Dr van Tiggelen. He believes that in many cases dementia can be cured, or at least helped. The elderly doctor who lost his patients cost the community $15 000 in three months. With appropriate management, van Tiggelen believes, the total should not have been more than $1000. Treatment and care for the man with the delusions cost $40 000 over two and a half years. It should have been $1000 or less if the hospital during the first week of admission had bothered to do a routine blood test, says van Tiggelen.

In his opinion, half the people in clinics and hospitals suffering from 'senile dementia of the Alzheimer type' should not be there. Early detection and early treatment can prevent further deterioration in a large number of people believed to be suffering from senile dementia, he says. Van Tiggelen, who is involved in research of chemical-induced brain damage, alcohol-related brain damage and senile dementia, has come across remarkable similarities in the chemistry of patients diagnosed as suffering from senile dementia of the Alzheimer type and patients suffering from brain damage presumably caused by excessive alcohol consumption. One of the similarities is the high incidence of depression in both groups. However, says van Tiggelen, it has been found by researchers that treatment with antidepressants rarely improves the condition of the senile demented patient.

Another similarity is found in the blood of patients with senile dementia of the Alzheimer type and in patients with chronic alcoholism — there is an imbalance in the trace elements copper and zinc. The ratio of copper and zinc in these patients, he says, is 'significantly different' from the ratio in 'normal' people and in sufferers from other types of dementia. Van Tiggelen suggests that the cause of zinc deficiency is due to an inadequate diet; or it can be caused by excessive excretion of zinc under the influence of alcohol or some other types of medication such as diuretics, which help a person to pass water. It is also possible, he says, that the imbalance develops because of hormonal changes, found in people with severe depression.

But he has found that the most interesting similarity between Alzheimer sufferers and alcohol brain-damaged patients is that in both groups there is a normal level of vitamin B_{12} in the blood but it is unusually low in fluid taken from the spine — fluid that has in fact passed through the brain.

'This low level of vitamin B_{12} is an indicator of an abnormally low level of vitamin B_{12} in brain tissue,' he says. 'It is widely known that deficiency of vitamin B_{12} in the central nervous system results in neurological and psychiatric symptoms, among them depression. But it also shows symptoms that can easily be confused with symptoms of early senility.'

Van Tiggelen and his fellow researchers believe that taking a measurement of vitamin B_{12} from the blood is not a good enough indication of the amount of vitamin B_{12} in the brain. But if it's in the blood, isn't it also in the brain? Not so, says van Tiggelen. Measurement of the vitamin in the cerebral fluid shows that this is not always the case. That being so, how can it be that an important nutrient for the brain like vitamin B_{12} is sufficiently available in blood but does not seem to get into the brain?

The cause, van Tiggelen suggests, is the imbalance between copper and zinc. Toxins, or poisons, such as a copper–zinc imbalance may impair the transport of vitamin B_{12} from blood to brain, while there are indications that the zinc deficiency upsets the brain's central noradrenergic system — the system that controls the blood flow in the brain and is responsible for the transport of nutrients from blood to brain. Researchers have found that when the noradrenergic system is not working properly, the transport of water, the most important nutrient for the brain, is impaired. Van Tiggelen believes that if one nutrient cannot get to the brain, others would also be failing. In his opinion, senile dementia of the Alzheimer type seems to be a condition resulting from the brain poisoning itself and being starved of nutrients. And he thinks that a number of conditions — genetic, nutritional, toxic and depressive — play an interacting role.

Genetic factors, he agrees, are, in a minority of people with Alzheimer's disease, undoubtedly involved. 'In its purest form, senile dementia of the Alzheimer type is probably a genetically determined disease,' he says. 'Depending on your genes, everyone will get it by the age of 120. In some people, the genetic penetrance is very strong; they will get it at a much younger age.' However, some people will develop early symptoms of Alzheimer's disease at a much younger age than determined by their genes because of the involvement of accelerating factors.

Nutritional elements can result in a zinc deficiency; an abnormally low zinc intake in elderly people's diets seems to be common. Zinc might be passed from the body, too, through alcohol and medication which remove fluids from the body. Prescribed drugs such as anti-epileptics and anti-rheumatics have been found to remove zinc from the body.

Toxic factors, says van Tiggelen, do play a role in the development of senile dementia-like conditions. Again, he names alcohol, but the blame can also be cast on chemicals such as industrial solvents, herbicides and pesticides.

Depression can also be linked to the development of dementia. Some depressive conditions can result in the abnormal production of hormones, which in turn can influence the copper–zinc balance in the body.

Based on the belief that dementia stems from these factors, van Tiggelen has drawn up a strategy to deal with patients with Alzheimer's disease, preferably those in a very early stage in order to prevent the development of irreversible changes in the brain. The idea, he says, is to recognise and treat as early as possible the accelerating factors. However, where genetic factors are solely involved — affecting only a minority of sufferers, in his opinion — every endeavour to treat or prevent the disease is illusory.

Among his suggestions for tackling the accelerating factors, he places great emphasis on health nutrition. It is vital to have a sufficient intake of water, probably the body's most important nutrient. And there should be an adequate intake of protein, fresh vegetables, fresh fruit and dietary fibre.

Alcohol, a potentially brain-poisoning chemical, should be avoided. On doctor's advice, medication should be reduced to the minimum required for the maintenance of the quality of life. Sedative drugs, hypnotics and other medications that go to the brain should be minimised. 'Great grandmother's hypnotic, a glass of hot milk with a spoon of honey and a banana, is just as effective as an hypnotic drug, as recent research indicates.'

Treatment and prevention of depression is also vitally important. 'It should be kept in mind that depression in old people presents frequently with a range of dementia symptoms,' says the doctor. 'Being depressed at old age, in the current Western psycho-social environment, possibly handicapped by physical and mental disabilities, is almost considered a normal condition. With increasing losses — safety, security, identity, role, status, territory, health, relations and so on — many old people need only one little additional event to develop their depressive reaction into a clear endogenous (self-produced) or vital depression. They lose interest, appetite, weight, sleep. They may become agitated and develop mental and cognitive impairment. Their ticket is ready: they are labelled as demented. No treatable causes are found and there appears to be a long history of cognitive impairment and memory problems — due to depression. Why remember things, when everything is useless and aimless? So the patient is labelled as suffering from Alzheimer's disease.

'Due to all the negative publicity around the disease, the doom of hopelessness, the atypically depressed patient is surrounded by people who do not have any expectations any more. It becomes a self-fulfilling prophecy. The biochemical changes in the brain, caused by the chronic depression, are adding up to the genetically determined decline of certain neuro-transmitter systems. Secondary changes due to effects on the blood–brain barrier occur, resulting finally in irreversible changes to the brain, fitting the neuropathology of Alzheimer's disease at the post-mortem five years later.'

He speculates that a person suffering from chronic depression at old age, showing significant cognitive impairment, sometimes complicated by an inability to express the depressed feelings, leads to hormonal changes. These changes could be an excessive production of steroid hormones, which in turn result in abnormalities in the copper–zinc ratio and affects the transport of nutrients from blood to brain. The result of these upsets, he believes, brings about a condition in the brain comparable with 'hibernation' of the brains in animals which sleep through the winter months. There is only one difference.

'When the environment threat in the animal disappears in spring, when sunlight is increased, temperature goes up, and cyclic hormonal changes occur in the hibernating animal. The supply of nutrients, in particular water, to the brain is restored and the animal wakes up from his "temporary senile dementia".

'Not so the human being. He has lost the capacity to modulate with changing circumstances. He is under an ongoing threat of the environment, maintaining his depression. Nobody has expectations; everyone and everything is adding to the existential environmental threat — no positive stimulation, no sunlight, no good nutrition. We are supplying potentially threatening medication and place him in a non-stimulating environment.

'In a number of patients diagnosed as "Alzheimer", we are overlooking an initially treatable depressive component.'

But van Tiggelen emphasises: 'Do not misunderstand me. I am not saying that Alzheimer's disease is curable. I agree that a minority of patients, currently diagnosed as Alzheimer, have developed the disease due to genetic factors. Nothing can be done about that; not in a way of curing or preventing the disease.

'What I am saying is that in a significant proportion of patients currently diagnosed as Alzheimer sufferers, additional and accelerating factors do play an important role, aggravating the disorder beyond the genetic impact.'

An oversimplified rule of thumb, he suggests, is this: every patient with dementia, who displays behavioural disturbances, hallucinates, has delusions, creates management problems, is basically suffering from depression. Only adequate treatment of his depression will reveal how severely demented he really is. Treatment should not be restricted to providing nutritional supplements and antidepressants; equally effective is the warm, sunny, optimistic, stimulating and communicating psycho-social approach.

Physical activity and anything that keeps the brain active should be encouraged. '"Live dangerously" is the best advice old people can get,' says van Tiggelen. 'Challenge your environment. Not everyone can become a Grey Panther, but interaction with your social surroundings, confirming the individuality and identity, is the best anti-depressant you can prescribe yourself. Be aware of people who want to "help" you — induced and learned helplessness is a guarantee to end up in a crippling nursing home, labelled as a senile dement with a co-existing depression.'

When the first symptoms of 'senile dementia' show themselves, get yourself on the following nutritional treatment, for a trial period of three months: 1 mg of vitamin B_{12} injected into a muscle once a week; one zinc supplement tablet every day. This treatment, van Tiggelen emphasises, does not produce any untoward side effects, but if after three months no beneficial effect is noticed, the treatment should be stopped. When improvement is noticed, treatment should continue daily with vitamin B complex, including vitamin B_{12}, in tablet form. And on alternate days zinc supplement tablets should be taken.

'This strategy cannot perform miracles. In some patients with progressed senile dementia, the damage is irreparable. In some patients the hereditary component cannot be treated. But we must be positive. We must fight against the doom of "institutionalised senile dementia". The vitamin B_{12} and zinc treatment may take longer to work for some and in others it may not work at all, but no harm is done in trying.

'I have been silenced by some of the incredible results we have seen, sometimes after six months of treatment. Not that the patient improved completely, but certainly we have noticed a considerably reduced amount of behavioural disturbances. There has been less agitation, less wandering, less aggression, less unhappiness. Most importantly, there has been no need to continue the use of sedatives or any type of hyponotic medication in severely demented patients. As for those seeking treatment in the early stages of senile dementia, we have seen remarkable improvements. People who were considered definitely on their way to an institution are still at home.'

Not surprisingly, van Tiggelen has angered the drug companies with his theories, for he vigorously fights against the use of medication. One Australian doctor observes: 'Dr van Tiggelen's theories about zinc and B_{12} deficiency are not mainstream medical ideas and it could be said that some of his good results stem more from enthusiasm and active, caring intervention than from any scientific, physical or chemical change. Most of the other ideas attributed to him are less controversial, but unfortunately not applied very often by treatment and care services elsewhere.'

Van Tiggelen accepts that more research has to be carried out to confirm his theories, but he strongly believes the public should be made aware of alternative methods of treatment.

'Pressure should be put on the "ivory tower" of medical research,' he maintains. 'At the moment, the main stimulation for research is coming from pharmaceutical industries which hand out grants and scholarships to conduct research into the effects of new drugs. I believe, however, there is tremendous scope for research into nutrition, but funds are lacking. If we leave treatment of senile dementia to the laboratory researchers, we may end up in a situation comparable to finding first the scientific and laboratory evidence for being hungry, before we are going to be allowed to eat.

'With a social and economic problem such as senile dementia, an epidemic of the next century, on our hands now, I think we may already be a bit late. When science and technology are getting to the point that they block and hamper creative imagination, they may be blocking progress and development. With the results of our treatment in our hands, I challenge the scientists to prove that I am wrong.'

Van Tiggelen, who works out of a clinic in Dandenong, near Melbourne, says that too often abnormal behaviour in a person over 80 is labelled as senility, and 'inadequate tools' are used to assess whether there really is brain damage. He says that there are, in fact, simple neurological examinations that have been known about since the turn of the century and which will give a doctor an indication as to whether there is any damage without having to resort to the expensive equipment of modern hospitals. Not only are these examinations cheaper, he says, but they help sort out the extent of complicating secondary and tertiary factors as well as the degree of treatable primary symptoms. In essence, the simple examinations give clues to the management of the person.

As an example, says van Tiggelen, an old person with brain damage might react adversely to medication. But by using simple examinations which test reflexes, a doctor can obtain clues as to which drugs to use.

To illustrate the investigation of primary symptoms, van Tiggelen refers to the case of Mrs Watson, an elderly woman with mild dementia living on her farm with her sheep, a cat and a dog. She managed reasonably well with the help of neighbours and meals-on-wheels visits. Suddenly, she became obsessed with the idea she was pregnant. Often she would be found wandering at night, trying to get herself to hospital because she maintained she was going to have a baby. At last, she was admitted to a country hospital with a nursery ward, and she was delighted to have babies around and looked forward to her own. But she could not wait and began wandering around during the night picking babies from their cots and nursing them. She was admitted to a psychiatric hospital for further management and care, and doctors believed her senile dementia was probably caused by sexual frustration early in life which was now manifested in her obsession with babies. A doctor began a thorough investigation and, out of curiosity, examined the pelvic region. There he found her 'baby'. She had a tennis-ball sized tumour in her vagina. What Mrs Watson was trying to say in her dementia, within her disturbed communication, was: 'Look, everybody, I've a feeling inside me which reminds me of the feeling I had 60 years ago when I had my first baby.'

Many doctors associate some mental abnormalities in the elderly with physical problems in the genital region. Early sexual frustrations, for example, might play on the mind, knotting the emotions to the point where the mind becomes deranged. But there are other physical conditions that can affect the balance of the mind — a prolapsed womb, growths and untreated infections. Van Tiggelen believes that searching for and finding these complaints can prevent the onset of irreversible dementia.

'Very often,' van Tiggelen says, 'the medical profession misses the message demented people are trying to put across. Too frequently, the talk of a patient with cognitive impairment due to dementia is discarded by those around saying "It's just dementia". That person is trying to communicate in his or her language. That we don't understand is as much our fault as theirs.'

Secondary symptoms are psychological, displayed when parts of a person's life starts to die. A heart attack patient who ends up in an intensive-care ward may cope psychologically with his changed physical condition. But how a person copes with a deteriorating brain function depends on his personality. If he has a memory problem, will he be aggressive and resentful about losing his memory? Or is he a well-balanced type who will just start writing things down? He might trigger off a defence mechanism, like denying he has a memory problem. Another person may be paranoid and accuse others of stealing his belongings because he can't remember where he put things. But the most common type of defence mechanism in a person who cannot cope with memory problems or brain failure is depression. Twenty per cent of old people living at home have depression; in institutions it soars to about 80 per cent.

Van Tiggelen recalls the case of a 55-year-old Yugoslav migrant living in Australia who was recovering from a stroke in a big hospital. Depression always follows a stroke and, says van Tiggelen, most people get over it 'unless doctors start interfering'. The hospital discovered Mr Kozak had high blood pressure and put him on medication. His depression worsened and communication problems started, so he was admitted to a nursing home. He worsened further, developing an agitated depression. Antidepressants were prescribed in fairly high doses together with medication for his agitation. Because of the damage caused by the stroke, the drugs had an adverse affect, and Mr Kozak developed Parkinson's disease. So the doctors prescribed anti-Parkinson drugs. These triggered off an acute confused state. As a result, Mr Kozak ran amok in the nursing home.

To quieten him, he was prescribed more drugs. However, the combined effect of the drugs caused an acute state of pseudodementia, as has been found in some types of brain damage. After a week of this treatment, van Tiggelen recalls, Mr Kozak was 'as mad as a rattlesnake' and ready to be certified to a mental health hospital. Yet today he is living quietly at home. 'How did this miracle occur? Another doctor took him off all his medication!'

Yet another type of condition, tertiary symptoms, is brought about by the social or physical environment. Symptoms may be produced when the patient's defence mechanisms come into play because he is being 'killed with kindness'. As van Tiggelen says:

'Neighbours, relatives and health providers, believing they are helping, focus on and emphasise his defects — emphasise the fact that there is something wrong. They tax his memory with needless questions. For someone with a memory problem, this sets off defence mechanisms and they either shut off completely or hit back.'

To show how physical surroundings can produce tertiary symptoms, van Tiggelen describes the case of an 84-year-old farmer who lived in the country for most of his life. When he developed mild dementia and started wandering on a nearby freeway, he was admitted to a psychogeriatric hospital built on modern lines and which included corridors with natural brick walls. On the farmer's property there had been only an outside toilet and when he wanted to urinate he would walk out and do it against the brick wall of the shed. When he was in hospital and saw the brick wall, his natural inclination was to urinate against it. This caused everyone to think he was completely incontinent and they started to devise medications that would help. What made matters worse was that the farmer's actions were infectious — five other men began urinating against the wall. 'The solution to this tertiary problem was quite simple,' says van Tiggelen. 'A clever nurse bought some wallpaper and paint and that was the end of the man's incontinence.'

He believes, then, that much unhappiness and expense can be prevented if an appropriate assessment is done early. Inadequate assessment can be detrimental and produce other symptoms. His case histories show that behaviour that demands help is brought about by disease or changes in the environment. These can be social, cultural, economical or ecological. Often the changes create more stress for the individual than his customary coping patterns can handle.

'Deviant behaviour — that is, behaviour that demands help — in the elderly, is never random or meaningless. The person is trying to communicate with his environment, trying to get across a scream for help. Unfortunately, the common answer is that the environment considers and treats the symptom as a disease, instead of listening to the message and seeking the real cause.'

Van Tiggelen says that if the help-demanding behaviour, the scream for help, is interpreted as a message referring to underlying causes, and if that triggers off an adequate assessment of what is still intact, this will lead to the person regaining his coping pattern.

'It will certainly help the person to find his equilibrium and maintain self-respect and will disclose what can be marshalled to improve the situation. In other words, an excessive and premature response to help-demanding behaviour, by doing things and providing immediate help for a person, weakens his capacity for coping.'

The psychogeriatrician believes that when an assessment is made, it should be started in the person's home. 'Trying to make this first assessment in an institution or out-patients clinic is like trying to study natural behaviour of the red kangaroo in a cage in your backyard.' Home assessment should reveal special problems in the environment, tensions in the family, and whether the person is being used as a scapegoat.

The next part of the assessment is a thorough physical examination by an experienced doctor, along with some blood tests. Van Tiggelen believes a good way to begin assessment is for a doctor to shake hands with the patient. This is not just a social nicety — it can be most instructive. It gives the doctor the chance to feel whether the skin is baby-like and smooth, which can give a reasonable indication about a person's nutritional condition, including some indication of vitamin deficiency. It is important for the doctor to find out what the patient knows of his disease history. Doctors tend to overlook a patient's opinion because 'it's only the opinion of a disturbed person'. A number of elderly people with brain failure do have problems expressing themselves, and the doctor has to try to understand their language. Van Tiggelen cites the case of a woman with brain damage who had a urinary infection. She could not express this, but related the pain to the cystitis she developed when she was newly married. She said: 'When I lie in bed in the middle of the night a stranger comes through the window and tries to have sexual intercourse with me and it is very painful.' What she was in fact describing was the pain of her urethritis and cystitis.

Van Tiggelen suggests that doctors look at the person's tongue, and if it is very red this would indicate deficiency in the vitamin B group or in iron. There is quite a bit of evidence, he says, to suggest that old people with a little brain damage might develop severe behavioural problems just because they have a latent iron deficiency, or because they have a latent vitamin or mineral deficiency, or a mild cardiac congestive failure which is treatable.

Malnutrition is a very common reason for disturbed behaviour in the elderly, and this should be picked up early. Dehydration is also frequently seen in old people, who can develop it within 24 hours of not taking sufficient fluid. The easiest way to check this — and relatives should be particularly aware — is to feel under the armpit. If it is wet and humid, the person is not dehydrated. If it is dry, the person needs fluid.

Next, says van Tiggelen, a superficial neurological examination can be carried out, not only by a professional neurologist, but by a GP or a community health nurse, by testing the reflexes. These tests include stroking the thumb with a pointed object, tapping the upper lip and tapping the tongue. A reaction by the muscles indicates problems in specific areas of the brain.

Following these tests comes the medical examination proper, where a doctor discovers any treatable and reversible disorders leading to disturbed behaviour. This should include a rectal and a pelvic examination. There should also be an adequate assessment of the senses, testing hearing, eyesight, smell and taste. Testing smell and taste can sometimes put doctors on the track of deficiencies such as zinc and magnesium. Poor hearing might easily result in withdrawn behaviour. Poor eyesight causes communication problems because people are not able to read or watch television and acquaint themselves with day-to-day affairs.

'What we should do,' says van Tiggelen, 'as soon as we are confronted with an elderly person with illness behaviour or "help-demanding" behaviour, whether he asks for home help, meals on wheels, laundry services, help with shopping or from a handyman, or for admission to a hostel, we should look at the underlying causes of this cry for help.'

However, he is adamant that wherever possible the elderly should be encouraged to live dangerously. 'Why should people who have made all their own decisions for 60 or 70 years suddenly, because they are that age, let other people decide for them? If an 84-year-old man, who had suffered a stroke, had two infarcts and has hypertension, wants to take a holiday from his suburban home and visit the Moulin Rouge, he might face a lot of family pressure advising him against it. But why shouldn't he go? If he does die there, he will die happy, rather than risk 10 years vegetating in front of a TV set in a nursing home? Risk is essential to life at any age, says van Tiggelen. We have to accept that some old people can live at risk and should accept that things can happen to them.

'If a demented old lady living in a dirty house with her pet cats is happy there and is not a danger to the environment, leave her. Don't be overprotective. She should have the right to finish her life as she wants. Our task is to support her as much as we can and as much as she will accept. Likewise, if after lots of good advice a person doesn't want to stay active and eat a balanced diet but prefers to stay in bed and eat fried chicken every day, take 10 tablets a day for the next 10 years, well, that's his decision. When he has been given the knowledge, the decision-making is up to him. Everyone lives at risk. A child in a playground or anyone travelling on the roads is at risk. Being at risk and under some stress and strain is a growth factor in everyday life, including the life of an old person.

'So for old people's psychological health, let them live dangerously. Let them take responsibility and do not overprotect them. What's more, you're allowed to dislike some of them: just admit it.'

Basically, he says, there is not much difference in the way we are talking about Alzheimer's disease now and leukaemia 30 years ago. 'Still, the five-year survival of leukaemia patients is going up every year, thanks to factors such as persistent research, early detection, early treatment, public awareness, availability of research money. Do we really have to wait 30 years before the medical profession in particular starts applying its mind in a similar way to senile dementia of the Alzheimer type, a disease which has a far bigger impact on the state of health and economy of the nation than any type of cancer?'

9

The burden of dementia

A person was talking about someone's loss of memory and resultant behaviour and exclaimed 'God forbid that this should happen to him or us'. I replied that God does not forbid and that it will happen to many of us and God might be the only one to help us then, since at present there are not many real helpers around with enough awareness to enjoy their helping.

— Lucia Raig, Sydney

The hands of the clock turn backwards. Skills disappear, speech becomes impaired, and families watch their loved ones slide into another dimension. They leave this world ... yet don't leave. The spirit departs; the body remains. Of all the assaults by nature on the human body, Alzheimer's disease is unquestionably the cruellest, for it erodes the whole being. The legacy for the families who mourn this living death is a human sack.

A well-known Australian publisher who had just had a baby was talking to one of her writers whose mother is an Alzheimer victim: 'My baby keeps me awake all night, crying and yelling, and even when I'm tired out during the day I still have to change and feed her. But I know it won't go on for years. Every week my baby is growing out of it. Every week your mother becomes more like a baby. I honestly don't know how you're going to manage.'

The sick family member asks for no love. Makes no demands for care. Yet those around him or her must devote all of their day and most of their night to the afflicted person. Sometimes it is under great sufferance, but they do it all the same, fighting back frustration, anger and fatigue. Like it or not, they must take on the role of cook, housekeeper, nurse and errand boy. It is a thankless task; the victims of this psychological death are just not aware of their carers. Nor does the public extend much sympathy. 'The spouse cannot mourn decently,' M.D. Lezak commented in the *Journal of Clinical Psychiatry*. 'Although he lost his mate as surely and permanently as if by death, since the familiar body remains, society neither recognises the spouse's grief, nor provides the support and comfort that surrounds those bereaved by death.'

Among the families who must bear the burden, many say that even most feared of diseases, cancer, would be kinder. As one notable neuropathologist, Dr Elias E. Manuelidis of Yale University School of Medicine, says, cancer allows the sufferer to retain his mental faculties and converse with his family up to, or virtually to, the end. His humanness goes with him there and then, but with Alzheimer's disease the spirit and soul has extracted itself possibly years earlier. The grieving cannot take place at that time because 'that time' is indiscernible. Neither could it end, for the family's loved one still has a second, physical, death to meet.

Because of the nature of the disease, early changes are often passed off as temporary aberrations by the victim and his family. Sufferers, confused by their failing intellectual abilities and fearing for their future, inevitably show signs of ongoing depression. Unfortunately, depression is not seen to be a serious malaise so it is easy for all to deny that anything is wrong. As the disease progresses, the victim's knowledge that his life is falling apart becomes blunted, but the family despairs more and more.

Says Barry Reisberge, a US gerontologist: 'The loss of a mind is too terrible for conscious contemplation. Dementia mercifully protects the individual against the horrible effects of this loss. Hence, it is the family member who must face the terrible reality of the illness process.'

In many cases, relatives will instinctively fight any suggestion that there is a problem. That their family member still *looks* all right helps them to explain away any curious behaviour as one of those things we all get up to from time to time as we get older. Initial denial also helps to soften the blow of reality. When they must finally accept that there is a problem, they have, in a way, been preparing themselves for it. But until that time arrives, the disease will have already been well set on its destructive course.

It is estimated that 75 per cent of mentally ill elderly people live with and are cared for by others in the community, usually a husband or wife or other close relative. These family members end up living a virtual mirror-image existence of the afflicted person: they must give up their job, they cannot go out to socialise, they avoid having friends in, they move through the day with little intellectual feedback — even basic conversation becomes difficult — and sleep little at night. At best, they must cope with endless repetition of the same question or statement and increasing forgetfulness. At worst, with hours coaxing the sufferer to eat and a constant cleaning up of faeces and urine.

A British woman whose father has a history of heart attacks describes the major problems he faces caring for his dementing wife: 'For the past six years my mother has suffered from Alzheimer's disease. The local authorities cannot offer any help to my father except in the form of a lady that calls once a week for two hours. My mother has hardly any recall at all, and cannot remember things that happened even yesterday.

'The doctor has done all he can, but the pressure on my father is immense. He has to bath her (she's 53), take her to the toilet, tell her what to wear each day, and also has to cook, clean and run, or try to run, his own business. He's losing weight, is becoming constantly depressed and needs someone or some organisation to turn to who understands this sometimes complex disease.

'My mother has an extremely limited vocabulary and sometimes doesn't even remember who I am — I'm her closest daughter. She didn't even know her own mother when they met for the first time in five years. My father's doctor has told me that if anything should happen to him, my mother would be put into a long-term mental hospital.'

Asked about their environment, care-givers say they feel imprisoned, trapped. Most say they suffer from emotional distress and nervous strain, accompanied by bouts of anger and impatience. One London man who was giving care told a researcher: 'Your own brain goes. You become so exhausted that you can't do any more.'

It is a major family problem — but it is more than that. Ahead lies a huge social dilemma. It is estimated that nearly 20 per cent of the population over 80 years old in the United States has moderate to severe dementia. Health workers are convinced that the social problems generated by Alzheimer's disease will increase; the very old will live longer and their care-givers, their younger relatives, will diminish with the trend towards shrinking birthrates. It is also thought that many career women will put jobs before family responsibilities and burdens.

US researchers Kane and Kane, after a study tour of six countries, reported: 'Seemingly, in each country visited, the family is considered to be the most constant support for the elderly individual... Daughters, often at great emotional and physical costs, continue to care for the parent unable to remain in his own home.'

A London husband wrote in a desperate letter to his local Alzheimer group: 'My wife has got worse in the past week. She has difficulty standing, walking and is unable to feed herself. I am feeling drained, but I have accepted the situation and hopefully will feel OK soon.'

The severe and almost intolerable burden shouldered by relatives who care for a mentally impaired elderly person is summed up in all its horror by a young English woman:

'My girlfriends are always asking me out to join them in their world. They go dancing, go to the cinema, have weekends away. That's their world. I can't talk to them about my life. It would make them physically sick. They just think I have to look after my elderly mother. I never ask them to come to the house. I make the excuse that my mother likes to be alone, and I never tell them what looking after mother really entails. It's like having a long chain that allows me to move around the house but not step outdoors. In one hand I have a sponge, in the other a wooden spoon. The spoon is for cooking — I seem to be at the stove for hours each day. The sponge is for mopping up urine because my mother will sit there and wet herself. Sometimes she does the other, too, and I've had to scrape it off from everywhere.

'At night, my mother won't sleep. She'll lie in bed and cry or groan or talk to herself. If I go in to check she is all right, I find that she's done something in the bed. At three o'clock in the morning I find myself stuffing soiled sheets into the bath to soak. My wrists and arms ache from dragging her backwards and forwards to the lavatory. I know that for my own sake I should put her into a home or a hospital, but there's the cost involved and I don't know if I could get her accepted anywhere. She's too far gone. It's not her fault, but sometimes I feel very bitter. I'm 39 and my mother is 72. She's had her life, and mine is burning away wiping up faeces. I look ten years older than I really am. I'm worried that when the opportunity at last comes for me to play, I'll be past it. That's my world.'

From London to Sydney, New York to Auckland, similar stories are told of similar households. Australian singer-actress Jeannie Lewis found she just couldn't cope with caring for her elderly mother who suffers from Alzheimer's disease, and after two years decided to place her in a nursing home. 'It was a case of her life or mine,' she says.

Jeannie's life with her mother and the decision to put her in an institution became the subject of Jeannie's show 'For a Dancer', written for the 1982 Adelaide Festival. Jeannie's problems began when she returned to Australia from South America and found that her mother was becoming unsure of herself and repeating things.

'The worst thing for her was that her mother had gone through the same thing, and I could see her getting tense and trying not to let anyone know what was happening. I think she realised exactly what she was facing, and was terrified.'

Two years later, after struggling to care for her mother, Jeannie realised she would have to put her into a home.

'In no other job are you expected to go 24 hours a day, month in, month out, year in, year out. I couldn't get anything done. It was selfish in a way. When I'd be trying to work she'd keep asking if I wanted cups of tea — I couldn't concentrate.'

A survey into the strain and anxiety felt by relatives of elderly patients at an Edinburgh day hospital — most of the patients were suffering from dementia — showed that nearly three-quarters of the relatives themselves were suffering from some form of psychiatric disorder. These pressures arise from problems in coping with a job, looking after children, holding up a marriage or just getting out at weekends. Anyone with moderate or severe dementia needs round-the-clock surveillance, a monumental burden for sons and daughters who are trying to get on with their own lives. There is a tendency for the task to fall on the shoulders of the daughters. Usually, by the time a parent has developed Alzheimer's disease, the daughters have married, are bringing up children and are 'around the house'. It falls upon them, then, to take on the task of care.

Because of the expectations of society and individual families, even women who have postponed marriage for career or travel reasons or simply for a sense of freedom find that they, ultimately, are drawn back into the family circle to care for their dementing parent. For her, at least temporarily, it is the end of ambition, goodbye career, and little hope of developing other relationships. 'I feel like I've been robbed,' says an Australian daughter who turned down marriage proposals for a life of freedom, only to end up caring for her dementing father. 'Some terrible thing has just come along and stolen my life.'

In the past, there was an even greater expectation that unmarried daughters should take on the responsibility of their ageing, demented parents. These unhappy spinsters are now elderly themselves, some with Alzheimer's disease. It is a tragic, vicious circle born out by the facts: in England and Wales in 1931, for every person over the age of 75 there were ten middle-aged people, but with the ratio steadily falling it will be down to three to one by 1991.

At first, many dementing people can manage at home reasonably well, as long as there is someone to keep an eye on them. Although this situation provides some relief for the family, children who live elsewhere must still make the daily or twice-daily visit to ensure that nothing has gone wrong. However, researchers in Britain have found that between a quarter and a third of all elderly people have no children, and nearly a half of all very elderly women live on their own — many having devoted *their* lives to their parents. Families either do not exist or are not available, and there comes a time when the already-overcrowded nursing homes or nursing services have to cope with yet another dementing person.

'Those families which can cope with their elderly dementing relatives carry a severe burden for all our benefit,' British psychiatrist Dr Marisa Silverman told her colleagues in a medical journal.

'They often come to the end of their tether because of regular difficulties such as sleep disturbance or dealing with faecal incontinence. Apart from relief facilities and prompt symptomatic treatment, they require opportunities to get out and also support and counselling for the marital and family difficulties that occur. Significant levels of anxiety and depression are noted in these relatives, but early identification of difficulties and response often maintains the patient with their family. Otherwise a crisis will occur after the point of final rejection has been reached by them.'

As Dr Silverman suggests, relatives who take on a caretaking role face disruption in their own family circle. As their dementing relative sinks further from them, changes occur in the way family members relate to one another. These disruptions are not restricted to husbands and wives, for like tentacles the problems reach out and touch every member of the family. A grandchild of a dementing elder might not be able to go to a soccer match on a Saturday any more because his father, who usually takes him, has to drive his mother to grandma's home so that she can cook lunch. A son and a cousin have to break up a business partnership because they have to share the task of care. A daughter-in-law lets her membership at the tennis club lapse because she cannot get down to the courts any more. Sometimes these changes of roles, resulting in various family members 'doing their stint' with the ill person, causes confusion in the sufferer himself. He may show his anger and abuse those who are trying to help, and this reaction will put further strain on what may already be taut relationships. Because the brunt of the caretaking usually falls upon the shoulders of the children — now middle-aged themselves — domestic troubles inevitably arise when a husband starts to count the cost of extra travel, or a wife, having raised her own family and seen them leave home on their careers, finds she now has to take on the role of parent once more, this time for her own parents.

One British geriatrician has calculated that for every demented patient in institutional care, there are five of equal or greater severity living at home. Of these, only 20 per cent are likely to be known to those who care for them regularly — the others will come to light only in a crisis. Nearly half of all psychiatric beds in Britain are occupied by the elderly demented, and one-third to a half of all local authority residential centres quote the same numbers. The problem will not get better. As the very old age group rises, the proportion of dementia sufferers will also go up.

Some struggling families blame the medical profession for creating a monster, a world where the demented elderly live on and on, where once they would have died without drugs to keep them going. George S. Robertson of the Department of Anaesthetics at Aberdeen's Royal Infirmary, referring to medical efforts to keep people alive even in the presence of advanced disease with limited hope, says this is seen as 'care based on the sanctity of life'. The fundamentals of this concept are largely based on religious belief, and this makes for considerable difficulty in understanding on the part of those who profess little or no religious conviction.

'The concept of the sanctity of life', says Robertson, 'has the corollary that many elderly patients and many relatives will be subjected to distress and indignity in circumstances where they might expect doctors to intervene on humanitarian grounds.

'This is not to suggest necessarily that the alternative to the sanctity of life approach is euthanasia. However, failure to suppress distressing symptoms in senile dementia, for example, may be seen as a dereliction of medical duty. Thus the main argument against the concept of the sanctity of life is that its logical and rigid application will be seen by many as an unseemly interference in the natural process of dying, with no quantifiable or meaningful objective.'

Question to a team of Australian specialists in Alzheimer's disease: What breaks can a carer give herself? How can she be realistic in her expectations of her own behaviour and that of the sick person?

Answer: What limits can relatives put on themselves in coping with a demented person? How much can they give of themselves? There *is* no answer for this. Each person is different and can give and cope to different extents. However, becoming a martyr does not help. You need some time for yourself. You need to make your life enjoyable. Some people cope by making the affected person the centre of their lives and devoting all their time and energy incessantly and selflessly. Often it is these people who find it most difficult to cope when the person dies and of course find it very hard to let go at any stage such as when the person requires nursing home placement. Sometimes the relative can wear himself or herself out, have a breakdown of some sort himself or herself, and then the problems of what to do with the demented person because you are in hospital or not able to cope are very great. Be realistic in what you can do and what you can expect. Just because a person has lucid movements or even lucid days does not mean that that is the level of functioning at which he or she can function always. These patches of improvement lead to false hopes and of course disillusionment.'

With the onset of Alzheimer's disease both victim and family enter a state of confusion. The afflicted person does not understand what is happening to him and the relatives are thrown into a situation with which they are unacquainted. And it's not a simple matter of learning to live with a 'set' condition, such as a case where a person loses a limb. After a time, both the victim and the family grow accustomed to that situation and learn how to cope with it. In a family where Alzheimer's disease has made its unwelcome entrance, constant adjustments have to be made as new problems arise and the personality of the afflicted person diminishes.

Researchers in Cleveland, Ohio, decided to find out the kinds of stress experienced by families, and conducted interviews with 600 groups who live with and care for their elders. Family stress, it was generally agreed, increased dramatically when the elder person suffered from advanced mental impairment, expecially when accompanied by behaviour problems and incontinence. It was found that adult married daughters with children were under the greatest stress. The overall suggestion was that the stress resulted from having to divide time between the ill relative and their own family and from receiving little help from other members of the family.

The Cleveland study, by researcher S. Walter Poulshock, found there appeared to be little in the way of effective family problem-solving methods to plan for and handle the crisis of caring for 'difficult' elders, most of whom were presumed to be suffering from Alzheimer's or related diseases. Among those suffering from great stress were the wives of men who had mental impairment, wives who were themselves getting on in years.

In Britain, researcher V. Wheatley conducted a survey among supporters of elderly people with a dementing illness living in the same household within an area covered by a south London social services department. He found a depressing situation.

'All the supporters in the sample under retirement age had suffered in varying degrees regarding employment,' Wheatley comments. 'Some had given up work to care for their relatives, and those who did manage to continue work had suffered numerous difficulties and disruptions.'

The 22-year-old great-great-granddaughter of an elderly woman — she was the only supporter — told the researcher: 'It was a terrible strain because I was all the time worrying about her, if she was all right. She'd go wandering off, outside the door, and the neighbours kept having to bring her back and were always ringing me at work. I had to keep taking time off, and they didn't like that, so it was getting too much for me. One day I just said to the manager: "I'm leaving".'

Wheatley reports that the symptoms of the actual illness which clearly caused the most distress were the mental abnormality and the faecal incontinence and, for those supporters with experience of it, wandering and abuse. The mother of one bachelor son was regularly both abusive and violent towards him. 'It's terrible, real gutter stuff, really upsets me,' the son said. 'And the crazy attacks — she never swore in her life, she was so clean — and the sexual fantasies, too. She is always being raped, she really believes it, then she'll go at me because I won't fight the chap who raped her.'

Says Wheatley: 'Although certain behaviour characteristics like stubbornness and restlessness did present difficulties, it was the mental deficits that were the most frequently mentioned, particularly those relating to the inability of the elderly person to communicate or to hold "sane" conversations. Also trying were the consequences of loss of short-term memory, and the frequent repetition by the elderly person of the same topic. In contrast to urinary incontinence, which all the supporters coped with without complaint, faecal incontinence was poorly tolerated and caused relatives considerable distress. One married daughter commented: "I have no idea of what she might do after finding it [faeces] in her handbag. I wonder what will happen next. One day I found it on the door handle, and several times on the handbasin. That's the very worst thing, quite the worst. I really hate that; I loathe it."'

The researcher found that all the supporters experienced considerable restrictions to their lives as a direct result of caring for their elderly relatives. Social activities were reduced, taking holidays was difficult, and anxiety was experienced daily over what the elderly person might be getting up to. One 68-year-old married person said: 'It's not a happy situation, is it? I mean, you sit like this all day. And just carrying trays of food. It's terrible just to go shopping and back again; it's a wasted life.'

Wheatley also came across the extraordinary case of an 85-year-old man, himself subject to dizzy spells and frequent falls, coping almost entirely alone looking after his 79-year-old wife who was doubly incontinent, wandered and caused havoc in the home. 'He had to do all their washing, cooking, shopping and housework, and although a district nurse visited once a week to wash the old lady (they had no bathroom) he had never been referred to the local social services department.'

In general, says the researcher, it appeared to be mainly chance that led to the supporters being in touch with social or health services.

'The supporters' lack of knowledge about the care system, even to the extent of being unable to identify who the workers were who visited them or where they came from, and their reluctance to criticise services, were disturbingly apparent.'

British psychogeriatrician Colin Godber is in accord with colleagues around the world that daughters and daughters-in-law generally take on the responsibility of caring for an aged relative, but he says they may have to weigh these roles up against their loyalties to their children, husbands and jobs. As dementia advances, he says, the need for supervision becomes almost constant, and where there are problems of restlessness, aggression or incontinence the burden is very heavy.

'The best way to avoid relatives being overwhelmed by the burden is to try to feed in what extra support is available as the load gets heavier — and to make sure that the load is in some way rendered intermittent,' says Godber. 'Often there are other relatives who can help, though one branch of the family is too often saddled with the whole load and becomes quite bitter about it.'

One woman, writing in a British national newspaper about the time spent looking after her mother, asks: 'What chance does a person have of returning to a good job if she wishes to take time off to nurse a dying patient? How many firms give paid leave for this purpose? I love my mother dearly, but I have no illusions about the cost of that love. Her comfort has been gained at the expense of my life. The only release is her death, and what do I do then? Who will employ a middle-aged woman, assuming that there's anything left of that woman to employ?'

Miriam Hirschfeld, from Tel Aviv University's School of Continuing Medical Education, interested to find out what influences a family to continue living with and caring for an old person with irreversible brain disease, conducted a survey of 30 families in an urban area of the western United States. She also wanted to find out what factors led a family to consider putting their dementing relative in an institution. As with other world-wide surveys she found that, in general, the middle-aged and older woman carried the burden of care for their ailing husband or parent. She did find, however, that in her particular investigation, 27 per cent of the caregivers were men who assumed full responsibility for the care of their often very impaired relative. All families had at least a minimal income, covering the cost of food, housing and medical expenses which are necessary for families to attempt to care for a severely impaired person in the home. Nearly half of the impaired group had trouble getting to the bathroom on time, 40 per cent needed 24-hour nursing care and supervision, 37 per cent tended to wander or get lost, and 27 per cent had a speech disorder or were completely unable to communicate verbally.

Ms Hirschfeld found the important factor determining whether a family should put a demented person in a home was not the degree of the illness but mutuality — the relationship between the healthy and the afflicted.

'In the face of immense problems posed by the impact of the decline itself, the implications of caring for a senile brain-diseased person and the difficulties rooted in the social environment, mutuality became *the* important variable,' she says.

Among those where mutuality was high, she met a family where the husband was severely physically and mentally impaired. His 68-year-old wife who fed him, bathed him and put him to bed at night said: 'He's a wonderful man. But now he is so confused and just like a child, a child that I love very much. Once in a while he still talks, but does not like to see me cry. He knows there's something wrong. We used to sing together and now he doesn't sing any more. Of course, I do everything for him, but I need him just as much as he needs me ...'

Another 'high mutuality' relationship was between a 66-year-old woman who lived with her 87-year-old mother. The elder woman was at times confused and 'crazy'. 'As long as my mother is not violent — and this is now taken care of by the medicine — we manage a good life together,' said the daughter. 'I will take care of her as long as she lives.'

In another group, where mutuality was low, families were so overwhelmed by the impact of the disease upon everyday life that the value they attached to the impaired person's continued presence was in jeopardy. They needed outside help in order to gain some free time and energy so they could see afresh a valued individual in the afflicted person. A son and daughter-in-law told Ms Hirschfeld about their mother:

'Right now we have no life; the whole atmosphere is so bad. Mother used to be a big help; we always lived together and it was perfect. She never had a mean streak in her, but now everything has become difficult. She forgets, leaves the water running, insists on cooking and can't do it any more, she constantly wants to feed us and is always accusing or blaming us for something. She doesn't realise that something is wrong with her. Now the biggest problem: when a little child doesn't act reasonably, you tell her or you put her in a corner and that's it. You can't do that to an old person. What are we going to do? We would like her to go to the Jewish home, but she'd resent it. It is hell if we do make her go and it is hell if we don't.'

A fourth group of people, who felt that their impaired family member had nothing to offer in any way to the everyday life of those around, would be relieved if the afflicted person could be well taken care of in an institution. Some people would be relieved by the relative's death. A 57-year-old man, who looked twenty years older, lived in a house with his wife, two sons and a daughter. His wife said:

'He was a wonderful father and the greatest husband. Our house was never dilapidated. He always wanted to work and then it started about five years ago when we noticed he would forget things ... The oldest son hasn't finished his thesis; he works as a night-watchman. The second boy dropped out of college and Anne is not doing anything; she was such a good student — now she just sits at home.'

The eldest son said: 'I used to love my father; I used to love to see him come through the door. Now when he comes, I hate it. It is like my emotions have changed. I hate to think that I hate my father now, but I just hate the disease he has. It's like I consider him dead three or four years ago ... He is like a symbol of how we live and waste away slowly. Sometimes I wish that he would die and I feel guilty for wishing that. Some things are worse than death.'

The bravery or the despair of the caretakers of the living dead is reflected in private homes around the world. At the onset of the disease, most families resolve to fight on, believing that once they adjust to a situation that cannot possibly get any worse, everything will be manageable. Time schedules will be able to be worked out, a cousin or a brother will be able to pop in and 'granny sit', and life will go on fairly much as normal. That is the illusion. For the situation does get worse. As dementia drags its victim down, it pulls the rest of the family with it. Little chores become major tasks; tiny obstacles become barriers. Friends begin to withdraw. The family finds itself isolated from the surrounding community and those everyday social interactions which are such an essential part of human existence.

Is this, then, to be the purpose in life? Waiting for the only release — death?

Can nothing bring relief?

Not really. But the burden of caring can be made a little easier. And any feelings of guilt, which invariably steal in to colour decisions that have to be made, soothed to an extent.

10

Caring: how to cope

In the absence of a cure, in the absence of a fairy godmother–doctor who can hand out pills and say 'Give these to your mother and she'll be well again next week', in the absence of brain transplants or even fresh nerve cell transplants, those who care for the dementing have to look at the alternatives. Thinking has to be geared to managing. How best to treat the individual without forcing on him 'learned helplessness'. How to incorporate him into your world rather than you sliding into his.

It is not difficult to see that improving the quality of life of a dementing person improves the quality of life of the carer. Health workers have found that those suffering from dementia are affected by their environment, so when the environment is adjusted to a point where the dementing person seems to calm down, the benefits are felt by the carers, too.

The quality of life can be upheld by helping the afflicted person cling for as long as possible to his or her skills. It has been found in hospitals caring for people with dementia that mental function has improved in some cases with the introduction of stimulating activities and physical exercise. Dementing people, it is widely accepted, do much better in their own environment, so helping them through familiar tasks in their own territory is seen by some psychogeriatricians as the only really effective way of slowing down the inevitable loss of everything. One British geriatrician says: 'Most practitioners are convinced of the benefits of maintaining people at home if at all possible, and these benefits probably include optimal stimulation of brain function.'

No one would pretend that this is the answer: give the dementing person something to do, and everything in the garden will be rosy. As the geriatrician adds: 'There comes a time when failure to cope produces such distress and anxiety that these emotions begin to reduce function below the optimum, and a vicious circle of increasing fear, failure and confusion is precipitated.'

However, stimulation can enable a victim of Alzheimer's disease to cling on to his skills for a longer period than if he were just allowed to drift away without any attempt to hold him back in this world. A 71-year-old northcountry woman in the United Kingdom told a social worker about her husband: 'He has been a very intelligent man and was an accountant for 43 years with the same firm and highly respected, given a wonderful retirement send-off in 1979. I think the fact that he had nothing to replace his work that he loved has got something to do with this brain complaint for he has deteriorated since retirement. I tried to get him interested in housework and helping with the washing and so on, but the only thing we do together is shopping ...'

Remembering Sir Martin Roth's comment that succumbing to Alzheimer's disease 'looks like death from boredom', health practitioners in the United States have been told to urge families to encourage their ill relatives to do whatever they still can do for themselves. Because the progression of the disease affects people in different ways, some may be able to do quite a lot for themselves up to five or more years after the diagnosis. The knowledge of how to add up may disappear, but a person may still be able to read. Another may be able to remember the words of old-time songs. Despite short-term memory loss, skills acquired *years before* can remain — cooking, playing the piano, tending the garden. So even though Alzheimer's disease cannot be cured, the outlook for all patients need not be so gloomy. They may be able to enjoy many more years of relative independence as long as they can be encouraged to do so.

A Bristol woman, whose sister-in-law is an Alzheimer victim, presents a frank, but encouraging, picture of life at home with her relative:

'She has been difficult at times, especially when we want her to do something, and will spend all day walking round and round the house or garden unless we persuade her to sit for a bit. There have been many things we've had to consider and work out, but at present she is on quite a good routine. She sleeps well and does feed herself. We can take her out and, because she is used to it, will join in a church service very happily, singing in her own way — she is accepted there. The family has adjusted well to her and I believe have benefited from having her here. Our young children love her but are not too wary to tease her and treat her like a friend. I'd just like to say that for almost 18 months now there has been little change in her condition. I feel this could be due to the busy home background — there's nearly always something going on.'

The United States Department of Health and Human Services advises doctors: 'Urge your patient's family not to ignore their loved one. Let them know the importance of a stimulating environment for the patient with Alzheimer's disease; but warn them of the fine line between stimulating and overwhelming. Remind them that Alzheimer's patients need the comfort of routine to get from day to day, but urge them to incorporate new sights and feelings into the routine. Encourage them to delegate simple chores to give their loved one a sense of usefulness and accomplishment. Tell the family to push the patient a little farther than is comfortable, occasionally setting tasks that are challenging without being frustrating. Coach a positive approach to the patient and his or her problems, but remind the family that the mental infirmity will become more obvious and more incapacitating with time, and may eventually lead to institutionalisation ... Throughout the illness bear in mind that the Alzheimer's victim remains first a human being, no matter how many intellectual faculties and cognitive skills may disappear.'

In all medical papers, in all official advice to doctors, in all suggestions whether they be from geriatricians or psychologists, the best that can be offered is an idea here, a possibility there, for holding on a little longer to skills that are under threat from Alzheimer's disease. No one is able to say how the illness can be reversed; until then, there is nothing the caring family can do but look towards maintaining the quality of life for themselves and their afflicted relative.

'I resent people saying she doesn't understand anything and doesn't know us,' says a Manchester daughter of her mother. 'Although she does talk mumbo jumbo, I hope she does understand how we love her.'

Depressing it may be that there is nothing to do but try to retain the quality of life for the sufferer, this is the cold fact that must be faced while scientists in laboratories around the world struggle on to find a way of beating the disease. While research continues, there is hope; and it is encouraging that because the disease has come to so much public attention more funds are becoming available for research. In the United States, $675 000 was granted to three schools of medicine for research into Alzheimer's disease. The grant, the largest from a private foundation for research in the disorder, came from the Commonwealth Fund, the president of which, Margaret E. Mahoney, borrowed medical specialists' descriptions and called the affliction 'the disease of the century'.

The first hurdle families must climb, then, is to face the problem at hand. Perhaps there has been a period of denial by the carer that there is anything wrong, but once the diagnosis has been made nothing will be achieved by hoping the afflicted person will get over it. However, this does not mean that you should not strive to maintain an optimistic and open outlook. Studies of cancer patients, for example, have shown that cheerful people are less susceptible to the disease. No one knows how the stricken family member will behave in future — whether he will go through spasms of anger or violence, or remain passive and be content to wander and sit.

Earlier chapters have shown that whatever path the Alzheimer person walks along in future is not of his choice; the brain, the control box, is slowly winding down and the body is getting out of control. Friends and distant relatives will sympathise but will not understand the hideousness of the problem.

'The effect of living with a much loved relative who suffers loss of dignity and all the other distressing symptoms of dementia can be catastrophic to a caring family,' says Mrs Morella Fisher, a London woman whose husband Lawrence was only 48 when his condition manifested itself. Now the founder of the British Alzheimer's Disease Society, she adds: 'Only someone who has actually experienced such a situation can really understand what it is like.'

This first hurdle — acceptance, facing up to the problems ahead — is sometimes difficult psychologically, but it can be helped by the whole family getting together and discussing how it should best be tackled. One of the first questions raised is whether the afflicted person should be told about the diagnosis. He or she will already be aware that something is wrong. Generally, doctors believe that all patients have a right to know about their diseases. This allows them to decide in advance how personal and family matters can be dealt with when they are no longer able to make decisions. However, with Alzheimer's disease patients, there may be greater problems in talking about it than there are in discussing other terminal illnesses.

Nancy Neveloff Dubler, an American legal and ethical expert on medical matters, raises the question of what is entailed in discussing the disease with a person who is at an early stage and experiencing some memory loss, word-finding difficulties or personality changes.

'Unquestionably, confronting this issue will be difficult for families and horrible for the patient,' she says. 'But is that patient not entitled to share the same process of mourning with his or her family as the dying cancer patient? If Alzheimer's disease is described as a "living death", shouldn't patients know about, ponder and face it to the best of their ability? Patients can then be assured of the same continued loving and supportive care promised to dying patients.'

Dr George Robertson of Aberdeen Royal Infirmary's Department of Anaesthetics believes that people should be encouraged to declare their own wishes in writing before reaching senility. By doing so, individuals may be able to spare themselves and their families the extremes of indignity which the elderly can suffer and inflict as a result of senile brain disease. Bearing in mind the dignity of afflicted people, he suggests that sedative drugs be administered to those who subject themselves to serious indignities such as persistent shouting or screaming. The 'double effect' of sedative drugs may clearly create the opportunity to allow dying without indignity, he says, but the primary intention should be the control of symptoms, not the hastening of death, just as the primary intention in terminal cancer is the control of pain. He suggests, then, that all people entering the last phase of life should sign a declaration along these lines:

'It is my express wish that, if beyond the age of, say, 65 years, I develop an acute or chronic cerebral illness which results in a substantial loss of dignity, and the opinions of two independent physicians indicate that my condition is unlikely to be reversible, any separate illness which may threaten my life should not be given active treatment. It is also my wish that if, during such cerebral illness, my condition deteriorates without reversible cause to the extent that my behaviour becomes violent, noisy or in other ways degrading, these symptoms should be controlled immediately by appropriate drug treatment regardless of the consequence upon my physical health.'

Once the family member and relatives know what has come upon them, it remains to give the demented person the best of life.

At the same time, it is vital to cling to your own self-esteem. If you start to be on the receiving end of criticism from other family members because of what you are doing or not doing or you are abused by the afflicted person, stand up for yourself.

An elderly Australian wife said in a letter to her Alzheimer support group: 'Last week, when having tea at our daughter's, mucus was dripping from my husband's nose and I told him to use a tissue. He said "I'm all right" so I said to my daughter "You tell him". She replied "It's your responsibility". So what can you do? If only my two children would understand, I would feel a lot better. Friends are all right, but it's one's own kith and kin that one longs for support from and they think I am belittling their father by treating him like I jolly well *have* to.'

You can answer your family however you wish, but you may have to be more tactful with your ill relative. This will be discussed later. The important thing is to respect yourself and what you are trying to do. Of course, a wrong turning will sometimes be taken, but do not feel guilty. Caring for a dementing person is very much a personal odyssey with solutions often arrived at in retrospect.

Ways of coping with the day-to-day problems are discussed in the next section, but one overriding factor is to try to ensure that the afflicted person remains in the environment he knows. Allowing close friends in to visit can help him retain a sense of the present, even though the changes in his brain will be trying to drag him into the past. He will begin to forget names — his friends should be warned about this so that they will not become upset and in turn distress the afflicted person. Other types of well-wishers in general should not be encouraged, for their visits will cause confusion. It has been shown time and again that any attempt to move the ill family member to surroundings that may seem much more pleasant to the carers will probably lead to a rejection of the new place and a flood of confusion. The rule of thumb should be 'Don't change a thing'. The only changes permissible are the faces of the carers, the family, who, if working well together as a task-sharing group will have worked out a shift system so they can all enjoy periods of relief. If afflicted people are to survive at home they must have an efficient carer or carers always in their presence. And they should be younger members of the family, not the husband or wife who will in most cases be getting on in years.

It has been found that early-stage Alzheimer sufferers who live alone or with their husband or wife usually have to go into an institution after twelve months, even if they receive house calls from qualified helpers. The rapidity of these victims' deterioration allows for little selectivity where nursing homes are concerned — they must go where there is room for them. They become another statistic, adding to the already strained nursing home resources. Worse than that, they invariably end up in an institution ill-equipped to serve up the amount of personal attention that dementia sufferers require.

The policy in many countries is to encourage families to keep their mentally ill at home for as long as possible to lessen the demand on institutions. Each case, of course, has to be treated on its merits — in some instances there is no alternative but to place an Alzheimer sufferer in an institution because he or she has no one to do the caring and the dangers at home are too immense. In Britain, there has been a steady growth in psychiatrists who deal with people with dementia, but there have been strong suggestions that their 'brief' should also include helping families and neighbours. The lack of real communication between the medical profession and the public is quite frightening. A good 'bedside manner' is often superficial as many professionals do not have the ability to touch the gut of the problem. Unfortunately, obtaining a university degree can also narrow the vision. As one carer cynically put it: 'The medical profession is geared to seeing that technology works and not in understanding the human psyche.'

P.H. Millard, Professor of Geriatric Medicine at St George's Hospital Medical School, UK, says the new breed of psychiatrists for the dementing must ensure that in defending the line of diminishing institutional resources they do not push people too far. 'The ultimate protest of someone who cannot cope any longer is murder.' And he points out that in developing a policy of home care for the demented, care must be shown to the carers.

Tom Arie, Professor of Health Care of the Elderly at the University of Nottingham, takes the same view. It is not so much a question of what the dementing person needs in the way of help but rather what are the most effective forms of help to families and other carers that will most enable them to carry the burden. 'It may be that our best investment is in what has come to be called "supporting the supporters" rather than in trying to support moderately or severely demented people who live alone and are likely to break down,' he says.

He sees this support as including all the traditional services of nursing, social work, home helps, meals-on-wheels, laundry services, day centres and 'granny sitters'. But Professor Arie concedes there are some patients for whom care in an institution is the only humane answer. And the staff to care for the growing numbers can be found, he believes, among those people who are now unemployed.

'Where these institutions are well run, where the staff are given real job satisfaction and a sense of worth — which includes proper support from the public and the administration, as well as proper leadership — and where the fabric and facilities are good, the care of the demented can be a challenging and rewarding job. The cost of enabling staff to move from the dole to employment in the caring professions has never been smaller and there is a real opportunity now. Furthermore, with the growth of automation and the likelihood of fewer work opportunities in the future, the business of caring will become a more and more important area of work opportunity.'

However, caring for the elderly mentally ill, even for the professionals in institutions and psychiatric hospitals, is not an easy task, according to Mr L.S. Christie, a former divisional nursing officer at Littlemore Hospital, Oxford.

'Those who have had little experience in coping with the elderly confused patient may not readily appreciate the task of a psychiatric nurse,' he says. 'It is a most demanding and exacting one, calling for considerable physical and mental stamina, patience, tolerance and expertise.'

He takes up the international cry for more beds, pointing out that the elderly mentally infirm represent a very large proportion of the in-patient population of psychiatric hospitals, and the demand for more beds and places shows little sign of declining.

'In the community, many families are attempting to cope with an elderly confused relative with limited support and resources, resulting in a situation where little comfort or hope is offered either to the confused person or his relatives. Social services day centres, hostels and private nursing homes are the alternatives to admission to hospital. But there may be constraints and limitations arising from the admissions policy — for example, the patient's mental or physical condition, behaviour pattern, mobility, degree of incontinence. Private nursing homes also lay down certain conditions even though the patient or the relatives may have the necessary finance to cover the scale of fees charged.'

Mr Christie says doctors and social workers are faced with the impossible task of trying to placate hard-pressed relatives. On the other hand, psychiatrists are reluctant to accept more patients for admission to hospital, because nurses are already hard-pressed. One of the offshoots of this problem is that old people's homes, the main purpose of which is to provide for a healthy elderly person an alternative to living alone or with an overworked family, are taking on the role of geriatric or psychogeriatric hospitals. A recent survey in Britain came out with the finding that in six old people's homes, half of the residents had symptoms of dementia. It is ironic that the original idea behind these institutions was security, comfort and a degree of refinement. Now, in a vast number, that sentiment has flown out of the window and we are left with depressing de-humanising boxes bulging with the demented waiting for the merciful release of death.

So until governments provide the backing for large numbers of special types of nursing homes and hundreds of thousands more staff are trained to work in them, relatives will be encouraged to take on the burden of care for as long as possible.

The immediate future will have its problems — between now and the end of the century, although the total number of people over the age of 65 will decrease, it is estimated there will be an increase of more than 50 per cent in the number of people over the age of 85.

Assuming you have had your family conference and you have made the decision, like most families, to 'give it a go' and look after your afflicted relative, where do you go from here? As suggested, you carry on about your day-to-day affairs as best you can, hope-fully with some form of rota system. If that is impossible and the burden falls upon one person, all is not lost. Try to discover what community reserves are available. Often, there are back-up ser-vices, but if you are completely unable to cope, a bed will always be found somewhere in a home or a hospital. There may be a waiting period, but if your needs are urgent, you will be given prime con-sideration in many instances. Making that final decision about whether to send the relative away or not can be a painful one, de-pending on previous relationships and so on. One of the added problems brought about by dementia is in attitudes — those who are physically most able to cope, such as healthy sons or sons-in-law, are reluctant to give up a good job to help look after an elderly incontinent relation whose behaviour is embarrassing and troublesome. Those who *aren't* able to cope, such as the elderly husband or wife of the afflicted person, accept the task more willingly. Research shows that young relatives can face placing their dementing family member in a home more readily than an older person. Those of the same generation are more able to identify with the situation — they know that they certainly wouldn't want to be 'put away', and a sense of guilt arises when they consider that alternative for their afflicted husband or wife.

To keep a dementing person in a nursing home is not cheap — although it has been found that first-rate home care can be just as expensive — and many families feel they have no alternative but to take on the task of care. As the number of demented increases around the world it has become more apparent that domestic carers need as much support as they can get.

As a result, support groups are now springing up in European countries, the United States and Australasia. Meetings are held and problems discussed, and it has been found to help a great deal when people find out that they are not alone. A typical support group was started in Britain's Cambridge area for relatives of patients confirmed as suffering from senile dementia. A psychologist takes the chair at each meeting, there is a twenty-minute talk on some aspect of dementia and the remainder of the one-hour meeting is taken up with open discussion. Present are psychiatric nurses, social workers and other medical experts who answer questions. Relatives attending for the first time are asked by a volunteer from the central team of experts whether he or she would like a home visit. In the home, the volunteer listens and watches for any problems that can be helped by other team members. Clinical psychologist Linda Powell-Proctor hopes the success of the Cambridge group will encourage people in other areas to form their own relatives' support groups: 'anyone willing to bring carers together would be responding to a current need,' she says.

In the United States a number of support groups have been started, one of the earliest being the Alzheimer Support Information Service Team (ASIST) which has 21 branches throughout Washington State. Mr Warren Easterly, a founding member, points out that often the family and friends are not aware of the problem facing the care-giver and the afflicted person until the disease has developed to an unmanageable phase. Lack of knowledge comes from statements from professionals, such as 'Your husband is senile' or 'Your wife has a memory problem' without an outline being given of the way a dementing person behaves. 'This causes the care-giver to minimise the full implications, leaving them unprepared for the anguish ahead,' says Mr Easterly.

Under ASIST — whose methods could be adopted by other communities — families, friends and professionals team together to work out the best way of making the task of care-giving easier. In the first meeting, a professional visitor asks how other family members have been able to accept the diagnosis, whether they think they can cope with caring, how their own health is and whether they will be able to adjust to a completely different life style. The care-giving husband will be told, if he hasn't already found out, he will become a housekeeper, cook, laundryman and eventually nurse; the care-giving wife will be warned that she will become the 'fixer' and treasurer.

One element of the illness which is given great consideration by ASIST is its devastating effects on an intimate relationship. As Mr Easterly says: 'There is no-one to talk, laugh or plan with; no-one on whom to vent frustration or share joy.' As a result, he says, the care-giver is encouraged to seek respite time for play, to express sexuality and to form other intimate relationships, while at the same time maintaining an affectionate commitment to the 'patient'. The care-giver, he says, is encouraged to stop 'dragging the lake for the moon'. For the Alzheimer family, the best system combines the concerned professional with caring supplied by family and any other members of the support system for limited periods of time.

'Intense personal involvement must be time-limited. Too often, the care-giver is isolated and destroyed by interminable caring and both care-giver and patient become a burden on society.'

ASIST's methods help families to keep their relative at home and functioning longer. There is less anguish and more growth in the ability of the care-giver and family to care for and understand the patient's decline.

Mr Easterly cites one case in which a daughter contacted the group and told them about her father, an Alzheimer patient, who had divorced and remarried before he was diagnosed as having the disease. ASIST was able to change a divided, guilt-ridden, trapped, confused, divorced family into a supportive coping group. The ex-wife, her four children and daughter-in-law began to give weekly periods of time for the care of the man, allowing him to remain at home. The present wife could continue her job, and outside help came for twenty hours a week.

As a contrast, Mr Easterly quotes a letter written by a woman who did not have the backing of a self-help group: 'My husband has been in a nursing home for 11 years. My money has all been spent and I will have to bring him home. I am only 61 years old and would like to do something with my life. But my children, my church and my town keep me tied to a corpse. Sometimes I feel like stealing away into the night for ever.'

This gives rise to an issue that individuals can only decide for themselves — whether they are foreshaking their marriage partner in seeking the companionship of a member of the opposite sex. You have to be brutally honest with yourself and ask whether you can cope with the scrutiny, gossip and alienation that often follows such a step. Let's face it, though, nothing brings more comfort than a balanced and caring relationship with someone. Unfortunately, many people do not wish the best for each other and prefer to see a lively, intelligent person go down with the ship. Anyone seen to be attempting to live life to the full attracts envy and resentment. And, curiously, not so much from others in a similar position as from family members and 'friends' who assume mantles of morality.

An English woman whose husband now shows no interest in her says: 'I started seeing someone else because my husband in a way deserted me. I married a particular man and finally found a stranger sharing my bed. This newcomer isn't the person I would chose to be with so I started a relationship with someone I wanted to be with. I don't feel bad about it. I just had to do it; just had to do it.'

An Australian woman, in a letter to a member of a support group said: '... I was beginning to wonder how I was going to face the future and what was in store for me, having to look after my husband who is no longer capable of giving and receiving love. I was despairing, when by chance I met up with an old acquaintance. We just started to talk about our lives and the things that had happened to us over the years since we saw each other last; our mutual friends and our families and ourselves. We both realised at that short meeting that we had an affinity that we could not allow ourselves to lose again. It was like putting on an old, comfortable sweater — it felt just right! We grew concerned about each other's well-being over a period of time and kept in touch by phone calls and brief meetings, and I grew to depend on these talks as something to look forward to, to lift me out of the doldrums. It was good to have a friend I could talk to and discuss my problems with, and also receive objective advice on problems that needed another opinion, and which the medical profession were not basically interested in ... He could always manage to make me laugh, even when my problems at home seemed insurmountable. He gave me a good feeling inside. He made me feel that I had more to give to life than just being a martyr to a sick person. With this inner strength, I have now become a whole person. I have taken up my hobbies again and feel that I can now tackle the world and that the future will now open up for me ...'

Those who volunteer to care for a dementing relative — or those who have the task thrust upon them by circumstance — do not have to sink. Support groups are springing up everywhere as public awareness of this disease of the twenty-first century spreads.

Often the support comes through hearing others talk about their problems and solutions. From such meetings, answers can be found to individual problems. Names and addresses of people willing to participate in a rota system of caring are exchanged. And for those who are at the frightening outset of taking on responsibilities, support groups help them to understand what is ahead — the personality changes, the day-to-day problems, the financial strain.

A British community nurse, Penny Hunt, emphasises the need for regular 'welfare' visits to a family caring for a dementing relative. 'This enables a sound relationship to be built up between the nurse and the family, ensuring a quick response in a crisis and relief arranged promptly if needed,' she says. 'When the family are aware that someone cares about their struggles, mental and physical, this can be the difference between their wanting to carry on or not.'

In Australia, the Alzheimer's Disease and Related Disorders Society (ADARDS), which has set up a care network, emphasises the need to make use of relatives and friends wherever possible to provide relief. Neighbours may well be able to keep an eye on the afflicted person while the carer goes shopping or has an afternoon off with friends. Sometimes relatives can help a particular carer to enjoy a holiday by taking on the job of caring themselves. And day centres might help a carer to continue a job before returning to care for the relative after hours. Temporary placement in nursing homes for a week to a month may provide just enough time for the carer to feel that he or she can cope for another six to eleven months.

'You will find', says ADARDS, 'that you are more able to care sympathetically and lovingly for the person if you are well looked after yourself — if you can get some time to "recharge your battery". You have seen the same problems with mothers who are totally with their babies and infants to the exclusion of any time for themselves. They become frazzled, irritable and produce more demanding and difficult babies, which then leads them to feel worse. Don't let yourself get into such a vicious cycle.'

That a dementing person needs grace-filled care is undeniable, however. As Bernard Isaacs, a British expert in medicines for the elderly, points out: 'Dementing people do notice. If they are treated sub-humanly, they behave sub-humanly. If they are treated humanly, not as "senile dements" but as people in their 70s — or even their 90s — with a long, active, useful life behind them but who have had the misfortune to develop brain failure, they respond humanly, often with good cheer, even with good sense and flashes of unexpected shrewdness. They can then be rewarding to work with, and can even, despite their brain failure, enjoy a happy old age.'

11

Helpful hints

As memory loss increases, disorientation, anxiety, restlessness, irritability and sleeplessness take over. They are conditions that need to be fully understood, or conflicts within and without the home will arise which will only add to the affected person's confusion and fears.

When the peculiarities of the mental disorder are recognised, the carer will be better able to handle the problems. The idea is to make life as streamlined as possible for the carer and his or her 'charge'. It would be wrong to suggest that with a few adjustments and a little understanding, all will be able to go on as normal. There will be days when the carer feels at the end of his or her tether. This chapter will help give you some ideas on how to live and cope with a dementing person.

Anger in the carer

'Nobody reacts with anger to diseases. If someone has a pain we give them medicine. If there is no medicine, we sympathise, we soothe in any way we know. But if someone simply forgets everything instantly, what is the medicine? How can we go on sympathising and soothing? And if someone accuses us of stealing, lying, whatever, how can we help reacting in our habitual way, as we have all our lives, with anger? And yet, this behaviour is only a disease.' — a Sydney daughter.

Your expectations of life have been shattered. Perhaps you are despondent, frustrated. You might be overcome with bitterness or even anger, for your husband, wife, a relative has been diagnosed as having dementia, possibly irreversible. The task of caring is yours. All your life you've worked hard, and you were looking forward to relaxing. Now it appears you'll have to struggle on for several more years. You know life won't get better.

Is it, as one woman asked her local support group, abnormal to get to the stage where you hate the person who is ill?

Sydney psychiatrist Henry Brodaty answers this typical question by pointing out that people have an enormous number of feelings about the illness and the person who is ill. There might be a denial and a numb phase where it is impossible to accept what is happening, he says. Then often there are times when you become very angry that the problem has hit your family. You might feel it is unfair for the person you love to suffer or that it is unfair for you to have to be put through this.

'You may wonder to yourself how he or she would act if the shoe were on the other foot. You may wonder about the past differences of opinion and feel bitter that now the burden of care has fallen on to you. You may well feel resentful about the loss of your freedom, loss of income, loss of opportunity to enjoy life or a number of other matters. You may also feel quite depressed, anxious about the future or generally sad. You may lose sleep with worry. It is because you can have all of these feelings that it is important to be able to share them with someone. Usually, the affected person was the one with whom you could share all of your worries and feelings but now this may not be possible,' says Dr Brodaty.

He suggests that feelings of anger and frustration can be lessened by talking to someone else who is close to you — or to those who are sympathetic to the problems involved, like others who have to care for an afflicted relative. A 'pool' of such people can be found at meetings of Alzheimer and related disorders societies.

There is nothing unusual about feeling angry. Even the most compassionate and relaxed of us react in moments of fear, love, happiness, sorrow and excitement; so when we are faced with a situation promising the worst our brains become alive with messages — 'deprived', 'why has it happened to me?', 'cheated' — and we respond accordingly.

We might look glum, we might weep incessantly, we might even strike out or, perhaps, not show anything at all, bottling it up inside where it hurts.

It is dangerous to nurture such emotions, because you might release them in a moment of uncontrollable rage on the dementing person who will be even more confused by your action. Initial

anger is understandable — your life henceforth is going to be reg-
ulated by cooking and washing and bathing and perhaps coping
with incontinence. As you become accustomed to this fact, your
anger will tend to dissipate but it might give way to dull resentment. In any case, make contact with your local Alzheimer and
related disorders group, or go to friends or relatives and talk it out
of your system. Talk is often the best cure for bad moods. One
woman closes the door on herself in her bedroom and screams for a
few seconds. 'I feel so much better afterwards. I've warned neighbours about it. I only hope I don't come face to face with an intrud-
er — no one will come to my aid!'

If you find yourself continually angry, try to identify the root of
the problem and then work on eliminating it. If, for example, your
relative tends to swoop things off shelves, put items out of reach. It
can in itself be frustrating, having to rearrange your books and
vases and putting them where they can't be appreciated. But at least
they will be safe, and you will undoubtedly grow accustomed to
seeing them in their new positions.

The former relationship between the dementing person and the
carer plays an important part in determining how they are likely to
ride out the future together. Some carers might experience anger as
a result of long-standing differences and problems in an association
or a marriage. One Australian woman, the youngest of three sisters,
caring for her father says:

'We never got along together, and still don't. But when he began
to lose his memory, I was the only one who would have him.
Actually, he hates living with me, but my sisters who were his
favourites have made no place in their lives for him and won't even
have him for a weekend. They say they can't stand the sight of him
dribbling and that he upsets the children. Somehow, the more he
slips away from reality the more aggressive he becomes towards
me, accusing me of the most awful things. It really upsets me and
sometimes I just don't know how much more I can take, but I can't
bear to think of him sitting waiting to die in a home.'

Then again, there are men and women who might have tolerated
ill treatment or neglect for many years. In an already vulnerable
state, they quite likely feel angry and resentful. For long the victims
of abuse, even cruelty, are they now to be slaves of a tangled mind?
Even if the personality changes and the sufferer becomes docile, it
does not wipe away years of anguish.

Whether the dementing person ought to be placed in a nursing home has to be an individual decision. But if the future is to harbour resentment and hatred, it would seem pointless and wasteful to spend more time under a heavy cloud, for carers face the very real danger of physical and mental collapse. The decision whether to institutionalise a dementia victim is never an easy one, nor can it be arrived at overnight. And no matter how bad a relationship might have been, it is often accompanied by enormous doses of guilt, a matter that will be dealt with later. But again, let's be realistic. For some people, an institution might be the only means of getting out of a relationship that has been endless and damaging.

There will be cases where families cannot afford nursing home placement. To avoid bureaucratic legal tangles and a lot of worry over what happens to possessions, consult a solicitor, preferably one who understands the people involved. The Alzheimer's Disease and Related Disorders Society (ADARDS) will also help to point you in the right direction.

Sometimes you'll be unable to put a finger on the exact source of your irritability and short-temperedness. There is not necessarily a single factor. It is more a build-up of circumstances: you haven't been able to get out of the house for days, weeks even, and your relative has been particularly difficult. You've had little time to yourself and nights of interrupted sleep. Nor is there any escape from the daily grind of domestic chores which always seem to take twice as long when you also have to contend with an Alzheimer victim. Then there are the endlessly repeated questions, the endless toileting. You are reminded by the mirror each day that time, precious time, is slipping away and with it, your dreams. And you watch the lines of tension and tiredness become etched on your face.

For younger women caring for victims of dementia, there is another reason why you may be unable to trace the source of anger — premenstrual tension. Only in recent years has this condition been accorded recognition, yet at its worst the inability of sufferers to control violent outbursts of rage have resulted in broken marriages, shattered lives and where eruptions have occurred outside the home — with a neighbour, for instance — lawsuits. PMT, as it is known, is only part of a whole syndrome or group of changes, physical and mental, which can begin from two to fourteen days before menstruation and are not relieved until the start of the woman's period. Mood change is common, giving rise to outbursts of irrational anger. Many women say they feel as though they are wound up to snapping point. It is not uncommon during this cycle for women to also experience depression, lethargy, swelling of the ankles and abdomen, vomiting, headaches, weight gain, swollen and painful breasts, acne and poor sleep.

Unfortunately, it is always when you look and feel your worst that you continually come up against people who question why you have chosen to care for your relative and who show little sensitivity to your need for someone to 'hear' how you feel. For you are not feeling sorry for yourself. In reality, it would be just wonderful to have someone put their arms around you as your mother once did when you hurt as a child. Remember that everyone, no matter that he or she might reach the age of 90, is still the child of someone and needs the comfort and love that a mother and father bring. Loneliness is devastating, and carers are often lonely, watching, ever waiting for someone who understands.

How do you beat these moments of despair? One suggestion, if the dementing person can be left alone, is to go for a brisk walk. Not only will you benefit from this exercise, but it will clear the cobwebs — at least for the moment. Or make yourself a cup of coffee and put your feet up. Call a relative or friend on the telephone and talk things over. Garden. Clean the carpet furiously ... anything to break the tension. One Melbourne woman refuses to buy a washing machine. She prefers instead to run around the corner to the laundromat when about to explode. Another woman takes a long cold shower and then makes herself up. 'I look in the mirror and see myself at my best. I'm cool and refreshed. It's as if I'm a completely different person. Looking different makes me feel different. What anger I had before is washed away down the drain hole.'

Don't reach for the brandy bottle and pour yourself a slug; that's just a way of clouding your own mind and not getting down to the root of the problem. Learning how to relax is difficult even for people who do not have the burden of an Alzheimer victim. Sometimes it is suggested you simply close your eyes and imagine a peaceful scene, cows grazing in a pasture, for instance. But this is easier said than done, and people who make these suggestions appear not to have had any practical experience of caring for an Alzheimer victim.

When near bursting point, it is all you can do to hold together, let alone take twenty minutes to envisage sun-kissed beaches and waving palms. You'll do more for yourself if you take off your shoes, sit in an armchair and put a damp flannel across your eyes for three or four minutes. Taking a shower and, for women, putting on make-up might help a great deal. You could also try putting on looser clothing. If there's time, go to the beautician or nip down to the local coffee lounge and read the morning paper or a chapter in a book. Some of these ideas might not be practical for everybody, but they can be adapted.

An Adelaide woman admits: 'I've rented a little flat all to myself. My husband is able to walk around at home and converse, and there are other members of my family around, so I feel perfectly justified in nipping off for a few hours and reading a book, making a cup of tea and luxuriating in my own solitude. I'm paying for freedom, yes, but thank God freedom can be bought.'

Do not, however, disregard the importance of relaxation. Not only does it help you keep your cool; it can add years to your life. But the art of relaxation must be practised. The British hypnotherapist David Shreeve says:

'You must be disciplined about it. Have a special time and a special place every day — probably the best time is at night, but not too close to bedtime so that you don't fall asleep.

'It takes about half an hour. Lie down. Think about the left foot, clench it and relax. Say out loud "my left foot is going limp". Think about it. Then do the right foot, the calves, thighs, stomach, chest, neck, face and scalp. The arms and the fingers. Then review. Go over tense areas again. Often the stomach, neck and shoulders need more attention. Put all unpleasant thoughts out of your head. Think only of pleasant things. This is not easy. It takes practice, but it is absolutely worth it. You will arise full of beans to work at night if needs be.'

A real difficulty when living with an Alzheimer sufferer is that whilst you must learn to have no expectations, you must continue to encourage your relative to have expectations of himself or herself. You might not expect thanks, you might not expect to have a trouble-free day or be able to go out when you wanted. But do not assume your relative will not respond to you. Dementia sufferers *can* respond. Much depends on how they are treated. Learn to separate yourself from the problems and not become swamped by them. If you feel frustrations welling up, it might help to take the afflicted person's hand and say something like: 'I'm going to try to help in every way I can. If you can help me in any way, I'd be grateful.'

You have now given yourself a responsibility so that duty to the task overwhelms all negative feelings. And you'll get a real boost if the afflicted person responds positively. Try to expel your frustrations as they occur — don't let them build up one on top of the other, because eventually they will only sour you.

As much as these suggestions will help in many cases, there will be readers who will consider them completely ineffective for their own particular desperate problems. And some of the problems are desperate. Consider the story told by Mrs Bartlett, a Sydney resident:

'We were living in England, my husband and my family, when we noticed my mother beginning to act a little strange. She started to lose her memory, there was no doubt about that, and she was generally confused. We had already decided to emigrate to Australia and I felt I couldn't leave my mother behind, behaving as she was. My husband was totally against her coming with us, but I had no choice. Moving to a new house in a new country in a different climate really confused my mother and she rapidly went downhill. The tensions in my family were terrible. My husband, already a heavy drinker, became totally reliant on the bottle and slipped into alcoholism.

'I had two young children who were screaming all day. The worse my mother got, the drunker my husband became and the more violent he became. I can't begin to tell of the number of hidings he's given me. They call Australia the Lucky Country — and I'm not blaming the country for what has happened to me — but since we arrived my life has disintegrated because of the terrible thing that happened to my mother. I found myself stuck at home with my mother who wandered everywhere, my children wouldn't leave me alone, and when my husband got home he'd open another bottle and take up where he'd left off before he went out. Now something even worse has happened. He told me that if I was going to have my mother in the house, he was going to have his, too. Now my mother-in-law has turned up and has moved in and expects me to wait on her, too. I don't know where it's going to end. I'm at the end of my tether. I honestly feel like killing myself.'

To ask Mrs Bartlett to lie down and think of green pastures or flat calm seas would be downright foolish. She has since been in touch with her local Alzheimer's disease support group who have been trying to help by talking over the problems with her. Even talking doesn't always help such severe cases. One problem in her family is compounded by another and another. Like others in such desperate situations, Mrs Bartlett feels the only way she can really solve her problems is to pack her bags and leave; walk out. But she does not want to leave her mother or her children. 'I'm trapped,' she bitterly concedes.

Anger and bitterness melt into one in many cases, and, psychiatrists admit, these feelings cannot always be talked away for good. But conversation with friends and supporters can help for a time. It is important, therefore, to maintain a good support system and not be left in a situation where you cannot ring anyone. Make sure, then, that you have a list of numbers. Above all, when you do feel waves of anger flooding over you, don't hold it in. Talk, walk, scream if you must. And don't feel guilty afterwards about your anger. You are only human — and anger is one of the emotions you have been given.

Often, the thoughtlessness of your own family members will drive you into a frenzy. They are swift to criticise, slow to help. Miss Evans, from the West of England, has been depressed and angered by the attitude of her father:

'My father was a very jealous man who clung to my mother throughout their married life. But when she got Alzheimer's disease she became my responsibility. The expectation that I should give up my life was assumed without a word being spoken. Whereas I had no objection to caring for my mother, it has been a difficult, thankless task. My father looms over me and never stops interfering. I can't do a thing right in his eyes. If it's a cold day and I close the window he says my mother needs air. If I open the window on a warm day he says she's in a draught. She'll get pneumonia one day, he told me when I opened up the windows, and it will be my fault when she dies. I know that when she eventually dies he'll see me as being responsible. Sometimes I think "Why do I have to put up with all this criticism?" But I'm doing it for my mother. It's the only thing that helps me get over the anger that roars up inside me whenever he starts his nit-picking.'

Another common source for anger is the medical profession. At the inaugural meeting of an Alzheimer group in New South Wales in 1982 some family members voiced anger against the profession, saying that many doctors either did not understand the disease or prescribed tranquillising drugs to calm the afflicted person down and left it at that. Psychiatrist Dr Brodaty, recalling that first meeting and the widespread dissatisfaction expressed against doctors, says: 'The lack of adequate service by the medical profession stems from a lack of knowledge, a lack of understanding of the problems, a defeatist attitude once a diagnosis is made, and some anger by relatives towards the medical profession for not being able to "cure" the affected person.' However, he adds, the anger over not being able to put the problem right is not the fault of doctors or other helping professionals.

Anger and frustration in the affected person

'I used to strain my ears to catch what my mother was whispering to herself about. When I would ask what she was saying, she would be overcome with confusion and shame and deny she was doing it. I used to remark, and now it fills me with horror, that talking to yourself is the first sign of madness. I wish I could turn back the clock. I would put my arms around her instead.' — a Melbourne daughter.

As Alzheimer's disease progresses, the sufferer will show varying degrees of anger and frustration. There is no doubt that in the early stages he is aware that reality is slipping away. Skills, familiar surroundings, words ... they all begin to recede, setting up fear and insecurity within the person. In his struggle to hold on to daylight, he reacts in a variety of ways. Often, he is overcome by restlessness, pacing aimlessly about the house, muttering, perhaps wringing his hands.

Frustration can turn to anger when the person begins to suffer delusions or hallucinates. He may believe you have stolen something from him when in fact he might have moved the item himself and now cannot remember where he placed it. Sometimes, there will appear to be no reason for his wrath. But it will almost certainly have something to do with the changing process occurring in the brain; the breakdown of the transmission system is resulting in confused messages which carry the afflicted person into another dimension where he sees things that aren't there in reality. You cannot prevent wrong impressions and you cannot stop feelings that are the result of them. What you can do is deal with emotions as they occur. To try to fight against them will only lead to further reactions — the person's confused brain has given him an immovable impression that something has happened, and for you to deny it will only cause conflict. Psychiatrists agree that a passive response will help to break down anger, but this is not to say that you must agree with any accusations levelled against you by the afflicted person.

If, for example, you are blamed for stealing a watch, don't respond with a harsh denial, and don't say that yes, you did take it. A 'neutral' answer is best, one that reassures the person and which also helps you to keep your own self-esteem. A good response would be along the lines of: 'Yes, your watch does seem to be missing. It must have somehow got misplaced. I'm sure if we hunt around, it will turn up somewhere.' Then have a look for the missing item. It it doesn't turn up, assure the person you'll have another look for it later or the following day. The point is to calm the person at the time with a reassuring answer, without admitting you're wrong. If you're in the right, remain in the right because you will not improve your relative's disease by admitting you're wrong — and you'll have lost a chunk of your self-worth.

Everyone suffering from Alzheimer's disease follows the same general, confused road, although they may wander on to byways that bring out individual differences in behaviour. Most experience some degree of frustration, and some do become angry and abusive, even violent. As a carer, it's important to ride it out and stay calm, trying to retain good humour. But it would be ladling out false hope to suggest that dealing with every angry reaction passively might eventually solve the problem. Confrontations between you and your relative can cause much pain and, if friends are visiting, embarrassment all round. There may be times when you are reduced to tears by the onslaught, particularly if your relative was a kindly, thoughtful person in the past. It is infuriating and it does wear you out, but try to look at the positive side of these expressions. Extreme though they may be, they *are* a reaction, showing somebody is in there. If a person is capable of evincing displeasure, he also has the ability to feel love, even if there might be problems in expressing it. Because of the brain's turmoil, anger and frustration manifest more readily than love, but that is not to say that deep inside the thickening layer of tangles and plaques, a storehouse of appreciation is not struggling to reach you.

View the emotion as a person's inbuilt reaction to changes over which he has no control. How angry he gets, and how frequently he expresses his wrath, may have something to do with the speed of the process of the disease, a theory yet to be confirmed. Some researchers think that the faster a person dements, the more exaggerated his emotions. But there is little doubt that restlessness, frustration, anger and violence are reactions against the brain's deterioration. Perhaps a subconscious awareness indicates that the natural run of life is being impaired; that restraints have been placed on memory and recognition, building up frustration to such an extent that a dam bursts. Usually the carer, the lifelong mate, is the scapegoat.

Another factor contributing to excessive emotional responses, a Sydney doctor explains, is 'disinhibition' due to damage to brain circuits which normally dampen or inhibit emotional responses. The result is the sufferer may have a 'short fuse' and may continue to be angry after the stimulus for the anger has passed. 'A related phenomenon', says the doctor, 'is "emotional lability" where sufferers, particularly those with multi-infarct dementia, can weep, laugh or be angry at the slightest provocation.'

As surely as scientists are unable to predict candidates for Alzheimer's disease, so it is impossible to say how individuals are likely to behave. Says psychiatrist Henry Brodaty: 'People with dementia have a tenuous grasp of what is happening around them. As they become more forgetful, they become more insecure. Some people then go to the extent of having to have everything ordered exactly to suit them, otherwise they become quite upset. Some people become quite suspicious about their relatives or spouses as they at some level sense their own failings and thereby feel quite inadequate. Sometimes an affected person may even become paranoid. Imagine, if you can, a world so difficult to comprehend because you are unable to remember what has happened, or what goes where, or what you should do or what words to say for something. You can now realise how frustrating it can be to have dementia.

'At times, then, a person with dementia might indeed have a tantrum, much as a very young child might do when frustrated by inability to control surroundings or to express thoughts or feelings of anger at a parent who is departing. However, when the tantrum is occurring in a middle-aged or elderly adult who is otherwise physically well, then this takes the form of violence.'

Dr Brodaty says the best way to cope with this violence is to try to prevent it in the first place by not arguing and by not putting too much stress on the person. There is no point in proving you can remember something better than the other person, for instance. You know you are right, and you will achieve nothing in the long term by proving it. Words sometimes get in the way of feelings, and a show of affection can be worth half an hour of argument and removes the problem at one stroke.

However, says the psychiatrist, a small degree of sedation is sometimes necessary if the person is becoming more violent. 'This may be only a phase of the illness; for example, when the person has the motivation and drive to do more but lacks the intellectual capacity to perform. If prevention has failed and the person does indeed become violent, it is probably best to let it pass and keep out of the way as much as possible. You would probably send a child who is having a tantrum to another room, but with an adult it might be easier if *you* went to another room. If can be difficult and frightening and it would be nice often to have someone around for support.'

Behaviour changes

Apart from a possible change in personality, the onset of Alzheimer's disease can bring out disturbing habits in your relative. He will get up in the middle of the night and wander. He might walk out into the street without any clothes on. Perhaps he'll urinate in a corner.

Some of the activities, while overall disturbing, can be seen in an amusing light by family members. 'My father', a New York man recalls, 'took the dog for a walk. He went two blocks, firmly gripping the lead. On opening the door when he got home he was greeted by the dog. He'd been down the street trailing an empty lead behind him.'

While the gradual changes in his brain have caused him to become forgetful, the afflicted person has also become a stranger in a strange world — a misfit. It's not even comparable to an educated person arriving in a totally foreign country where customs are different. Such a person soon learns to adapt. For the Alzheimer victim, the changing conditions brought about by the disease are like being transported to a different dimension where the social proprieties of everyday life do not exist. He might not see a chair as something to sit on but as a place to urinate. Place mats on the table might be for eating. Clothes, he might recall, are for wearing but how to put them on is a different matter.

Researchers have found that those going through the early stages of Alzheimer's disease tend to behave more 'oddly' towards the end of the day. It has been suggested this is because their slowing brain has become even more tired, or because they cannot see as clearly. Whatever the reasons, it will be found that as the disease progresses the different behaviour patterns reach back into the day until at last there is no time when the afflicted person is not on a different plane.

Unlike any other disease, dementia manifests itself through behaviour. Victims do not acquire strange growths or suffer extreme pain or break out in high fevers. Its onset is so gradual that its hold is already established before anything unusual is admitted. Unfortunately, there is no means at present of pinpointing a potential victim and taking steps to prevent the disease from taking hold. We have to wait for unusual behaviour patterns to set in before we can even be suspicious that it has developed. Then there is usually another waiting period of some six months before specialists can make a comparison with earlier behaviour and attempt a diagnosis. The afflicted person might make some comment himself at first such as 'I did a silly thing today — I read the newspaper for ten minutes before I realised it was a week old.' Harmless enough. You'll laugh, he'll look sheepish. He might do something equally 'silly' the next day, but he will probably not mention it this time because he might think it peculiar that he has started to do these things. He'll start to cover up. If he's late home because he couldn't remember where he lived he might say he was delayed at the office. But eventually you'll realise that something is very wrong. He might, just might, say he's losing his memory a little, but it will be an unusual confession. He'll know something is going wrong, but he won't really be able to put his finger on it unless he's aware of Alzheimer's disease. He certainly won't want to believe he is going through the early stages of this devastating affliction, and he will possibly deny it even to himself.

A Sydney woman says: 'They sent my husband home from work one day, telling him to have a long rest. He was in charge of a new adding machine. If you pushed the wrong button a bell would ring. He didn't want them to know he was capable of making mistakes and they found him poised like a statue, his fingers hovering over the keys. He stayed there like that for several minutes. That's when they decided he needed a holiday. They said they'd see him in a week or so. That was three years ago. He was 45 years of age. He never went back. Never will go back.'

So what do you do when you suspect something is happening to your relative? Perhaps he has always had an amiable personality and telling him that you think he is going through some sort of mental change might not be daunting. Or perhaps you face a stranger displaying characteristics not in evidence previously. An Australian wife recalls: 'There were hysterical outbreaks at our son, with never any rational quiet talks with him. Never instructing, always picking. Never discussing, always picking. Never helping, always picking.'

At some stage, whatever reaction you expect, it is only fair on your relative to tell him that he is undergoing a change. Sit down quietly, have some music on perhaps, and tell him the truth: you suspect something is wrong and perhaps a proper diagnosis should be made. One psychiatrist suggests explaining that a part of the person is ageing more rapidly than the rest of him, and although it is a disease of memory everything else is intact and there are ways of compensating for the loss of memory.

Not everyone behaves the same when they are in the grip of dementia, but general patterns are noticeable. Victims — for that is what they are — follow their relatives closely around the house, they might become suddenly quite paranoid, make unreasonable demands, make accusations that articles have been stolen from them. They'll be listless at times, aggressive, depressed, hide objects or shift them from one place to another, be unable to find the bathroom. There is no known way of permanently stopping these traits. The carer has to realise that they are all part of the disease. Patience and understanding on the part of the carer is of prime importance. Without it, both the sufferer and the carer will slide downhill together.

Wandering

News item, Melbourne, 23 February 1984: 'A big police search was mounted today for a 67-year-old woman who wandered from her home. Her husband, who was away visiting a doctor, told police his wife was in a confused state. The couple live in an outer Melbourne suburb, and there is concern that the woman has wandered into the bush towards the Yarra River.'

One of the big problems with dementia is that it impels the sufferer to wander. The afflicted person will get up in the middle of the night, like a sleepwalker and perhaps leave the house. He will turn into this street, walk down that road, follow a back lane, until he is completely lost. He might wander around the house and head down the road to the local shop during the daylight hours, become disorientated and head for home — in the wrong direction. Perhaps the person's restlessness is due to frustration, for it is as though these sufferers are searching for something that eludes them. Families report that wandering seems more prevalent at night, and this added confusion might be tied in with other behaviour changes brought about by the brain slowing down at the end of the day. No one knows what the exact reasons are; we can only accept that those suffering from dementia are inclined to wander and can be a danger to themselves. They might walk past the kitchen stove and absent-mindedly knock over a boiling saucepan. They might walk out of the front door and cross the road without looking for traffic. They could wander on to someone's property at night and be attacked by a neighbour who mistakenly believes it's a burglar. An Alzheimer victim might step on to a bus without having the money to pay for the fare and become embroiled in an argument with the conductor.

A Welsh farmer's wife: 'I was very worried. I hadn't seen Hugh for several hours and told the police that he was missing again. They'd brought him home several times before after people had rung about a stranger standing in their garden or a man acting oddly in the shopping centre. But this time they had had no such report. He was missing overnight and I was convinced he had had an accident and no one had found him. They finally found him, in Cardiff, at a fair. He had got on the big wheel and was going round and round. He'd given the man a five pound note and because he couldn't change it then he said he'd give Hugh the change when the ride was over. But Hugh stayed in the chair so they thought he wanted to go round again. It went on like that for ages until one of the men thought they had better tell a St John's Ambulance man. He realised something was wrong and took Hugh to the ambulance station, from where they rang me. They'd found my name and address in one of Hugh's pockets.'

Unless you can keep a constant eye on your dementing relative during the day and be sure that there is no means of him getting out of the house at night, you should see that he carries identification with him at all times. His name, your name and address on a card in his wallet would be fine if you could be sure he would always take his wallet with him or not misplace it. But of course it never works that way. You could put cards in all his pockets in all his clothes, but he might pick them out and throw them away. Short of tattooing your telephone number on his forearm — one American woman seriously considered that — the most reliable means of ensuring your relative will be returned home is to have his name and address engraved on an identification bracelet, which cannot be removed. Various countries have different types of bracelets, but an enquiry at a local jewellery store might help you find what you are looking for.

In some countries, such as the United States, a medical bracelet is available on which a special 24-hour telephone number is engraved. Individual families can decide what is best — for example, if their afflicted relative never leaves the house without putting on his hat, the answer would be to engrave a telephone number inside the hat as well. It might be stating the obvious, but if you have a relative with dementia, it's essential that you are on the telephone. If financial reasons prevent this, contact your local welfare group or your Alzheimer's support circle and explain the problem. If your need is genuine, help will come. Good Samaritans are still to be found.

Trying to prevent your relative from wandering can become a Catch-22 situation. If you lock the doors and hide the key, the person becomes more agitated and confused when he can't get out, particularly at night. In the early stages of dementia, the person is less likely to be a danger to himself — he still remembers to look for traffic before crossing the road, for example. But as his judgement becomes increasingly impaired, real danger arises. Only individual families can decide how their relative reacts to being locked in during the night; however, locked doors are the kindest means of dealing with wandering. Put the bolt at the bottom of the door where it is less likely to be seen. It's highly unlikely the dementing person will go to the stage of smashing a window to get out, although that has not been unknown. Another idea is to hang a bell from the top of the door so that if it is opened during the night, you'll be woken.

Some nursing homes, because of shortage of staff and patients' wandering tendencies, strap people into chairs or beds. It is a drastic measure, guaranteed to raise their temper. Restrained against his will, the patient becomes more angry and confused and, unless medication is administered, is likely to begin shouting and screaming as well. But to be fair, if he is not strapped in and wanders off and is lost or injured in some way, the nursing home receives the wrath of the relative.

Question to ADARDS, Sydney: Is there any way of dealing with a wanderer other than with a restrainer?

Answer: The person with dementia who wanders is another difficult problem. There are no good facilities for the wandering dement other than to be placed in a locked ward. The latter requires committal under the Mental Health Act and is a step that most families seek to avoid. Nursing homes cannot be locked by law, yet people with dementia may wander on to streets and get lost or even run over. It would be ideal to have nursing homes with large grounds and gates which were difficult to undo, but these are few and far between. Sometimes wandering, though it occurs, isn't really a problem if the person is adequately labelled; for example, a large notice stuck to his dressing gown. Helpful passers-by will usually return the wanderer after a pleasant stroll. To me, restrainers seem barbaric.

That nursing homes with large grounds and secure gates are rare is true at the moment, but establishments could follow the example set by the Senior Citizens' Department of the Regional Municipality of Niagara, Canada. They operate long-term care facilities for the elderly, some 17 per cent of whom are what they describe as 'mentally frail'. The department has set up 'therapeutic parks' after considering such questions as: How could parks change confused and wandering behaviour to more functional and reality-oriented behaviour? How effective could an external surrounding be for our mentally frail residents? Is it possible for such parks to modify or stabilise behaviour? They went ahead and built, putting in special gardens with gazebos, walkways and features such as old-fashioned water pumps and ancient horse-drawn buggies. And the fences, instead of being brick or wire, were made of lattice-work and cedar logs. The residents of the nursing homes attached to the parks were able to walk as much as they liked without becoming lost. The Municipality reports:

'There is no doubt in anyone's mind that the parks have caused considerable improvement in our mentally frail residents' ability to function in this unit. The parks have raised the residents' self-esteem, stabilised their overall behaviour and to some extent brought them back to an awareness of their present surroundings. Moreover, these changes have indicated a heightened appreciation of the outdoors, and increased mobility. This, in turn, appears to be increasing sociability and enriching daily life experiences.'

The concept could be minimised and changes introduced to your own home environment to encourage your relative not to wander. Do you have an uninspiring back garden with a broken-down gate through which your relative always 'escapes'? If in the early stages of dementia, perhaps the person could be encouraged to help tidy up the garden, improve the landscaping, do something about fixing up the back fence to make it presentable. It might be cruelly compared to a man building the walls of his own prison, but the idea is to take the burden of constant watching away from you, while providing a pleasant environment for your relative — an environment that he might enjoy staying in or working in.

While wandering at night is more common than during the day, families who have moved addresses after dementia has been diagnosed agree their relative becomes more confused and tries to leave the new house, almost like a cat trying to return to its own territory. The person is, of course, searching for familiar surroundings. When he knows his territory, he feels secure; away from it, his agitation increases. Some families have had success in setting up their relative's room in exactly the same way as in the previous address. There, he finds the security that he might be searching for in his wanderings.

Is your relative getting enough exercise under your supervision? His wandering might not be due to lack of security but because his body feels a *need* to move around. Some families have found that if they take their relative for a daily walk, it helps to lessen the agitation. Setting up a routine — such as walking to the local shopping centre and having coffee — can help to give your relative some purpose to the day, and if he should wander off from the house you might know where to look. 'My mother', says a Swiss woman, 'always walks to the school she used to attend nearly 60 years ago. It's about two kilometres from the house and every second or third day she has this compulsion to walk back there, along the same road from the same house that she walked as a child. It's the only place she goes to. Sometimes she has gone right into the class room and the teacher has taken her to the staff room to wait for me to come and collect her.'

It's a good idea to alert your local shopkeepers, police station and neighbours about your relative's confused state and give them your telephone number. That, in addition to an identification bracelet or cards in his pocket with your phone number on them, will ensure you are informed about his whereabouts. People rarely become lost for ever. However, you will experience additional trauma with a wandering relative if you live near water, a wooded area or in the country. In metropolitan areas, shopkeepers or passers-by will notice if someone is acting strangely and perhaps tell a policeman. As more people become aware of dementia and less frightened of it, there will be a greater community response when someone wanders off.

Disorientation and safety in the home

As confusion worsens, even a home that has been lived in for many years becomes hard to negotiate. This adds to the insecurity and frustration of the sufferer. It helps, then, to set up a house in such a way that it aids the afflicted person to know where everything is. Put his personal belongings — photographs, old trophies — in view. Always put any items you use back in the same place. The emphasis is on familiarity.

This is not to suggest you put up huge signs with arrows pointing in every direction, but signs on doors can help a great deal. For example, put a notice on the bathroom door reading BATHROOM.

And, if possible, include an illustration of a bath or a toilet. Painting the bathroom door in a distinctive colour might also help the person identify that particular room. Wherever there are switches or taps, put signs beside them indicating which is which. On a gas cooker, for instance, a small sign reading FRONT BURNER or REAR BURNER might help. An arrow pointing to the left or right instead of the words left or right might help some confused people. Without some sign on the cooker, a confused person might turn on a tap, fail to ignite the burner he thinks he has turned on, and walk away, leaving the gas on.

If you're going to take your relative for a walk, don't just dress him up and lead him out. Tell him where you're going and how long you expect to be away. Point out neighbours' houses, and remind him of the people who live there. The idea is not so much to help him remember the names of neighbours but to stimulate his brain.

Always put his clothes in the same place. The same goes for newspapers and magazines. Don't move the furniture around. And at night keep the bathroom light on and perhaps the light in the hall so your relative can find the way without fumbling for switches or falling over things in the dark. Anything that creates a hazard should be moved. Don't leave any sharp utensils lying around — keep them in a locked drawer. Things such as electric irons and power tools should also be kept out of sight and reach. And one important consideration is the temperature of the water in the tap. Dementing people are not always able to distinguish between extremely hot water and cold, and they can scald themselves severely.

In several countries, what is known as a reality orientation programme has been found to be successful in giving a dementing person a sense of security. Although it was introduced nearly twenty years ago, the technique did not catch on until the late 1970s. It requires some effort on the part of both the carer and the afflicted person, but it has been found to stimulate the person and lessen his frustrations. Under the reality orientation technique, you, the carer, continually remind the person of who he is, what time it is, and what is happening in his surroundings. Linda Powell-Proctor, a psychologist at Cambridge's Fulbourn Hospital, Great Britain, who advocates the programme, suggests that instead of silently escorting a person to the table for lunch, the carer says something like: 'John, it's now one o'clock and time for lunch. Shall we go to the dining table and sit down?' The carer is encouraged to speak clearly to his or her 'charge' as often as possible, using direct eye contact and touch to maintain their attention. The idea is to bring the affected person back to reality by constantly reminding him of the practicalities of everyday life. But don't treat the person like a child — the ideas is to talk to him simply, but on his level.

What safety in the house comes down to is plain common sense. If something is dangerous, move it. If things are hard to find, make them accessible. If the door to every room looks the same, put signs on them. The time will come when your relative will not read the signs, and you will have to take on a greater role of helping him about the house. You have to remember that your relative is as susceptible as a child. Keep your best china out of reach, wipe up any spilled water in case he slips and, of course, lock away anything poisonous that could be consumed. You even have to remember such things as the washing-up liquid or laundry detergent. Just because it tastes dreadful doesn't stop a dementing person putting it in his mouth.

You will have to make a decision whether you want to live in a house that is suited to your own comforts or practical for your dementing relative. To maintain it as you want it will be a constant battle. The crockery you like to display will possibly get broken, your plants will be shredded, lamps knocked over. You don't have to live in Bleak House to make life easier for the afflicted person, but you will have to do some rearranging. And you'll be earning some peace of mind.

Driving a car

Don't let him. Anyone with dementia should not be in charge of a vehicle. Sell the car or hide the keys. Remove the rotor arm or pull the leads from the spark plugs. If an altercation develops because you won't let him drive, give him the keys and let him try to start it. If you have 'fixed' it, he'll soon give up.

If you need a car for shopping, tell him the car has broken down and keep it parked in another street. If you have to go somewhere by car with the relative, go by cab or get a friend to drive you. Should you need the vehicle to drive your relative frequently, change your present car for another, keep that parked elsewhere, and when you take it to the house to pick him up, tell him a friend has loaned it to you on the condition that only you drive it. If you constantly use the vehicle and you keep telling him the same story, he'll become accustomed to it and will not protest. Sometimes you just have to tell white lies for his safety and the safety of others.

Incontinence

Despite your clearly labelled bathroom door, you'll find one day that your relative has been unable to find it and has either wet or soiled his clothes. It is an unfortunate aspect of dementing illnesses that finally so much of the brain is affected that victims end up unable to control their bladders or bowels or both.

Emptying the system of its waste products is a natural function. Most of the problems arise because we are schooled to regard them as secret activities which we joke about or use cute terms to describe. As well, these are traditionally very personal functions so that when someone else witnesses an 'accident' and has to help in the cleaning up, it causes a great deal of embarrassment and distress. It is an affront to the individual's dignity.

Bearing this in mind, when faced with a situation where a person either urinates or defecates in his clothes, try to clean up without fuss and try not to chastise him for having done so. You'll find if you treat it as 'much ado about nothing', it eventually becomes no more than a routine exercise. And irritation and frustation will blow through you and not raise your blood pressure.

Loss of bladder control usually starts first. But before jumping to the conclusion that it is permanent, explore why it might be happening. For instance, an infection in the urinary tract or the bladder can cause incontinence, as can other medical problems. So, too, can certain medication. And is the person really wetting himself, or 'leaking' as often happens with exertion or nervousness? Do not disregard psychological causes; fear and insecurity may also need to be taken into account. Be thorough in your investigations as there is the chance that incontinence can be controlled to some extent at the outset.

Does he wet himself before medication or before having a bath?

If the medicine is distasteful or bathing traumatic, he may be showing his displeasure by letting everything flow. You may need to change his medicine or bathe him after he has used the toilet. If your relative tends to lose control of his bladder during the night, you could try limiting the amount of liquid he takes during the evening, although it is important he has an adequate amount to drink during the day. Perhaps his bedroom is too far away from the bathroom. You could help him by leaving a light on at night and if the two rooms are separated by a hallway, leave one on there as well. Or you could purchase a commode for his room.

No matter how clearly marked the bathroom door is, no matter that you have lights blazing, accidents will happen. For the person will want to go to the toilet, get up, ... and lose his way. In his desperation, any corner, any room, a flower pot, a walk-in cupboard, will do. Even if it happens over and over again, try to remain patient and see the positive side — he *was* trying to get to the toilet, and anger will only confuse and shame him so that his behaviour worsens.

It's essential that you invest in a washing machine because you will be faced with a daily pile of soiled clothing and sheets. If you can't afford one, contact your local welfare society or council department and explain the problem. Some Alzheimer support groups are now making general funds available from a central kitty to help desperate families. Even if you have to pay off the washing machine by the week, having it in the house is going to save you hours of dealing with soiled, smelly clothes and bedding.

In the early stages of incontinence you might notice that your relative goes at certain times — for example, as soon as he gets up or just after breakfast. If there is any regularity, take the person to the toilet at about that time. You might have to pull down his clothing as a signal to him to 'go'. Turning on a bathroom tap sometimes prompts a person to urinate.

If you are feeding your relative adequate amounts of roughage and giving him regular exercise, you can train him to open his bowels at about the same time each day. Don't worry, though, if this doesn't happen. Metabolisms vary, and so long as his stool is not hard or pellet-like, a good bowel movement once every three days is all right. Anything longer than that and you should begin checking what you are feeding him and whether he is getting enough water to drink. Too many people rely on tea and coffee, rather than plain water. Try not to regard squeezing fresh citrus juice as being too much trouble. It might make your relative want to urinate more frequently, but it will help regulate his bowels and so make it easier for you. It goes without saying that laxatives are best used only in dire emergencies; even chronic constipation will respond eventually to diet and exercise.

Anything to do with bladders and bowels can be a distasteful subject for many people, but with a dementing person it's a problem that has to be faced. And remember, you are not alone. There are hundreds of thousands of families who are having to deal with the same processes of nature. At first, even pulling down someone's underwear might be an unpleasant task. Having to wipe a bottom might be beyond comprehension. The very thought of it might make you want to run through the front door and never return. Do not feel bad about such a desire. After all, if you're suddenly faced with caring for a dementing, formerly straight-laced parent, it is shattering to be responsible for keeping genitals clean and wiping a bottom. Many people find that after a few times it's not so bad. Try to see it as unpleasant for only a short while. There's always plenty of soap and water around for you to wash yourself should things get a little untidy. But if you really can't face it, you'll have to arrange for a nurse to call each morning and hope the timing is right.

Because a relative loses personal control, it doesn't mean that clothing, chairs and mattress have to be ruined. There are effective ways of preventing this. Absorbent pads that work in the same way as nappies are available from all chemists and can be worn inside the normal underwear or inside special plastic pants that can hold one or more pads. They are disposable, and when soiled they can be wrapped in newspaper and put in the garbage or the incinerator.

You can also obtain special absorbent sheets to place under the person at night so you can be assured he is not lying in a wet bed. Most department stores also stock mattress protectors. Some are claimed to be odourproof, but it is advisable to spray them from time to time with a freshener spray. Some protectors are not totally waterproof and a sheet of plastic should be used beneath them.

Smaller versions of the absorbent sheets are available to fit chair seats. If you have a loved antique chair, the obvious course is to put it in a place where the person cannot use it. If common sense prevails, you can continue to surround yourself with beautiful things.

The environment you create will also help your relative. Encourage him to use a particular chair and tell him it's his, for his personal use. A cheap plastic tablecloth cut to size can be laid out over it and is effective in preventing any dampness getting through to the surface of the chair if he wets. And you can put fabric over it if it looks unsightly. You could even make a special removable cover to match your other furniture. Although incontinence is a burden for the carer, it's not so bad knowing that what is available for babies can also be purchased for adults.

You might not even have to worry much about soiled nappies or pads if you establish a routine of taking the person to the toilet. Most families find that taking them along every two hours works reasonably well, although there will be times when the person won't go in the toilet — and waits until he is guided back to his chair. He isn't being perverse; he might simply have got his timing wrong, or decided that this chair was a much more comfortable place to sit than the toilet seat. If this happens frequently, try putting foam rubber on the toilet seat and remarking how comfortable it is to sit there.

If the person is not able to communicate to you verbally that he wants to go while sitting in the lounge room, there might be signs that you will be able to read. He might 'tut-tut' or wriggle. Sometimes it means that you're just too late, but often it is a signal that they want to use the lavatory.

No one would pretend that coping with incontinence, particularly bowel incontinence, is one of the more enviable vocations of life. Some families find that when bowel incontinence begins, it is time to look towards nursing home placement.

Bathing and grooming

If old people, or people suffering any illness, mental or physical, are not kept clean, their skin tends to give off a sickly-sweet odour. In this society, cleanliness and lack of smell are important for social acceptance. So it is necessary for both the carer and his or her charge that every effort is made to keep a person suffering from dementia well groomed at all times. This is not easy and is time-consuming, but the rewards rub off on you as well.

At first, the affected person will be able to manage his own bathing, providing you're around to turn on the water tap to the right temperature and to ensure that he doesn't fiddle with the taps during his bath or shower. Whether you use a shower or a bath obviously depends on what facilities you have in your home, but if you're prepared to install either, both have advantages and disadvantages. A shower is quicker, probably more efficient, but a bath is safer — the person can't fall down — and is possibly less traumatic. It is certainly easier to persuade a person to walk into a shower than it is to slide into a bath. Either way, the water will soothe and relax him. Never leave a confused person alone in a bath. If he's well advanced into Alzheimer's disease, he might have to be lifted in and out. The very old, say over 75, mostly should not be bathed every day because their skin has less oils than a younger person and they are more likely to develop dermatitis, especially in winter or in cold climates where the air is drier.

If you prefer, there is a specially made bath seat available, which rests on the edges of the bath and allows the person to sit with his legs in the water. A rubber hose attached to the taps enables the person to be washed. Alternatively, you can purchase a special seat for the shower. If it's too expensive, buy a small cheap chair from a department store, ensure that it is fitted with rubber on the ends of the legs and put that in the shower. A suitable type is a chair with a wire seat and back with a plastic coating.

Should you be concerned about your relative being alone in the shower, change into a bathing suit and get in too. It might not be a case of 'you scrub my back, I'll scrub yours', but you'll save a lot of time and frustration. The idea is to keep wash time simple. If your relative resists, trying combing his hair first and telling him how well groomed he looks. Help him shave — an electric razor is a must — and then lead him to the water. If he still resists, you will probably have to resort to sponging him down with a flannel. Once he's wet, getting him into the shower or bath might not be so difficult, but if he still refuses you at least know that he's reasonably clean. It's important that the genitals are cleaned and also the areas under arms and breasts. Use talcum powder or a similar powder after ensuring that the skin is perfectly dry. Then you can tell the person how clean he looks and how nice he smells. In many cases the person will associate bathing with feeling good and not with some kind of torture.

You must always be present when electric razors or hair driers are in use. Preferably, razors and driers should be used in the bed-room, away from water. A plugged-in razor which falls into a filled wash basin will give a fatal shock if someone reaches in to pluck it out. Many people have died as a result of a plugged-in drier falling into their bath. As an extra precaution in the bathroom, use plastic mugs, not glass, for storage of toothbrushes or for drinking. As for teeth cleaning, you will probably have to measure out the right quantity of toothpaste on to the brush and actually carry out the cleaning for a confused person. And make sure you do it, because a neglected mouth can lead to terrible problems in the latter stages of dementia.

Therapeutic bathing

Have you ever thought of a bath as having a purpose other than to clean the body? With the addition of certain herbs and plant es-sences it can be extremely relaxing and soporific, or energising and circulation-building. Many ancient cultures realised this and de-veloped their social life and institutions around group bathing and splendid bath houses. Which is not to suggest that you introduce your relative to a communal pond, but if you have time to try some of the following ideas they could be of great benefit to someone suffering dementia.

Most of the herbs used grow readily in the garden or in a pot on the windowsill. Even the dried variety in your kitchen cupboard are all right. You might even be able to enlist the aid of your relative in planning a herb garden, which will eventually become the source of your supply.

The quickest and easiest way to prepare the herbs is to put them in an oval, stainless steel, hinged tea-making ball, available from most department stores, attach it to the hot water tap in the bath, and let the water flush the essences through. Remember that although you need the hot water to draw off the properties of the herbs, *never* soak your relative (or yourself, for that matter) in very hot water, as it de-energises the body and irritates sensitive skins and thread veins.

Although this method is the simplest, the only way to get the most out of any herb is to spend time in the kitchen infusing or decocting (boiling down). An infusion is made as you would a strong pot of tea, using about 1 pint (600 mL) of boiling water to two to four tablespoons of leaves or flowers, depending on how strong you want it. Do not boil the herb. Pour the boiling water over the herb and let it steep, covered, for at the very least fifteen minutes. The longer you leave the 'brew', the stronger and more valuable its properties. For best results, put it aside for up to three hours, but no longer. And use only crockery, glass or ceramic pots or stainless steel. Never use aluminium or non-stick pans.

Alternatively, combine the herbs with cold milk. It extracts the essences without heat. Use in a proportion of one tablespoon per cup of cold milk and leave covered for up to two hours.

When using bark, roots or seeds, they will have to be boiled for a minimum of 30 minutes. Again, don't use aluminium or non-stick pots.

Another method of drawing off the properties of herbs is through extraction with alcohol. This, however, requires planning — the process takes two weeks. Pour half a cup of alcohol into a jar, and add herbs until the container is filled. After steeping for a week, strain, then add more leaves and repeat the process. At the end of the second week, pour the liquid through a cheesecloth or nylon strainer. You will know the preparation is ready when the alcohol retains the scent of the herbs. You can make the extract go further by adding a quarter of a teaspoon of simple tincture of benzoin and a quarter of a teaspoon of boric acid powder, each being dissolved in three tablespoons of witchhazel.

It's a good idea to keep a non-slip rubber mat on the bottom of the bath and large rough towels nearby, as a vigorous rub down afterwards is just as much of a tonic. The simplest routine, and very effective, doesn't even require herbs: add a cup of apple cider vinegar to the water or, for a really stimulating dip, dilute the vinegar with eight parts of water and rub it into the body before getting in. Because apple cider vinegar balances the acid content of the skin, it alleviates tiredness and relieves itching, flaking or drying of the skin. Another mixture good for circulation is a combination of 500 g of Epsom salts, 500 g of magnesium chloride, and eucalyptus, pine or mint extract oil. This should be added to the bath water. Should you wish to use pine needles you have gathered yourself, boil them for 30 minutes; treat eucalypt leaves as you would tea, but steep them for 25 minutes. Both pine needles and eucalypt leaves are particularly helpful where body aches and stiffening joints are a problem.

Some common healing herbs are:

Chamomile Soothing, healing and cleansing. Good for insect bites. Also makes a calming tea if your relative is restless at night. Use fresh leaves and flowers or dried flowers.

Comfrey Remarkable for all-round healing. Particularly useful with rheumatic, arthritic joints. Leaves make a marvellous poultice for all kinds of sores, burns, swellings. A strong infusion made from the leaves can be used in the bath water — for external use only, of course.

Marigold (calendula) An aid for healing body scars, sores. Good for varicose veins and thread veins.

Mint Aromatic and soothing. Good for skin eruptions or heat rash.

Garlic and leek Both excellent skin tonics with healing properties for sores, cuts and ulcers.

Linden (lime) and nettle Contain a compound similar to natural hormones. Nettles contain vitamins A and D.

Dandelion Can be combined with nettle for a nourishing bath.

Other calming and healing herbs that can be used individually or together are: rosemary, thyme, parsley, sage, fennel and blackberry leaves. Popular and easily obtainable aromatic herbs to add to the bath are lemon and orange blossom, jasmine, lavender, roses and mint. You can also enrich the bath water by sprinkling rose petals in the bath as it fills. Choose the petals from one of the old-fashioned sweet-smelling variety. It goes without saying, of course, that plants must not have been sprayed with any insecticide.

And if you have no time at all, you can always sprinkle a few drops of oil into the bath water to keep the skin soft and supple; try sunflower, sesame, avocado, apricot, coconut or almond oil.

Communication

The degree to which language is lost varies from person to person. Some dementia sufferers reach a stage where they cannot speak at all, but do not assume this will necessarily happen to your relative. This breakdown in communication is due to the progressive failure of the person's neurotransmission system: messages passing in and out of the brain are interrupted and distorted. Hence, the endless repetition of a question or sentence.

A dementing person will not remember his words of a moment

before. He is not being deliberately irritating. He just cannot recall asking the question in the first place. Often, too, you will find him using the wrong words for things, or you will have to call his name three or four times to get his attention. Whatever his response, try not to frustrate him more by flying off the handle, and if he does not attend at all, give him a hug and get on with what you were about to do anyway.

Sometimes the description a dementing person applies to certain objects is almost the right word, but not quite. He might say 'kip' instead of 'cup' or 'telemission' instead of 'television'. Sometimes, instead of using the correct word for an object, he'll refer to it as a 'thingmijig' or a 'what-do-you-call-it'. It doesn't do any harm to remind someone about the word they are looking for, providing it's done tactfully. The important thing is that although the person's mental faculties are declining, he should not be talked down to. Remember, you might have to repeat something because he hasn't grasped it the first time — or he will have immediately forgotten what you have just said. If you want to speak to him, call his name first to get his attention. Then speak clearly and slowly and ask if he understands. Lower your vocal pitch; higher tones imply anger and tension, and that will make him immediately less able to cope.

He might reply 'Of course I understand' when in fact he hasn't quite got what you have said. There is no way of beating this. Misunderstandings and repetitions are factors you will have to learn to live with. But you might be able to learn through non-vocal signs and from his eyes whether he has appreciated some of it.

Even if you are encouraged by a conversation you have in the morning, a discussion in the afternoon might fill you with despair because your relative has become much more fractured and distant. One of the characteristics of progressive dementia is the fading in and fading out of lucidity. Often, the person will start to say something, then leave the topic dangling. Take advantage of his lucid moments to talk to him. Discuss the news you've read in the paper — if you've had a chance to read the newspaper! — or on the radio. Such topics might help to stimulate the brain cells that are transmitting relatively well. If you try to engage your relative in conversation when he is on a low communication level it will only confuse him and frustrate you. Of course, if he talks to you, you should reply. Try to remember that when another person is present, don't talk about your relative as if he isn't in the room. Include him in the conversation, so that instead of saying something like 'John seems to prefer tea to coffee nowadays', say 'John seems to prefer tea to coffee nowadays. Don't you, John? Perhaps we'll have some soon, what do you think?' Conversations such as these include the dementing person and also give him a chance to say something. There is the consideration, of course, that drawing your relative into a conversation focuses attention on him in the presence of others, which might add to his confusion or frustration. You must try to develop an awareness so that if something causes him much distress, you can drop it or steer in another direction.

Unfortunately, we have grown too dependent on verbal skills. Remember, there are many ways to reach out, be understood and understand through body language and so maintain communication with even the most severely impaired sufferers. Despite loss of ability to speak and coordinate movement, they remain acutely aware of non-verbal signals. Try to become sensitive to your relative's expressions, no matter how slight. Watch hand, body, eye and head movements. And be patient when waiting for a response — remember, your instructions have a tangled web to get through. You'll be surprised at how much you can actually pass on and the feedback you receive. For instance, if you remain calm and cheerful, your body will transmit this to a restless sufferer, and he will eventually quieten down himself. Smile at him, touch him, tell him he looks well. This doesn't mean fussing over him 24 hours a day, but let him know you are near by if he needs you.

If your relative has lost his speech as a result of a stroke, he should come under the care of a speech therapist as soon as he is well enough. Many people have learned to speak again when there seemed little hope.

Money cannot buy the high quality of care that a cheerful and loving relative can give. Just hugging him, holding his hand, getting him to sit with you instead of popping him out of the way to bed every night, will bring him comfort and reassurance.

Legal matters

If a relative becomes so mentally impaired that his ability to sign his own name or know what he is signing is lost, problems of ownership of property and finances will arise. A son or daughter struggling financially might find trouble gaining access to his or her dementing parent's resources even if an inheritance has already been promised. And should a person die having not made a will, relatives might find themselves embroiled in a legal battle with the government. Legal affairs can be a source of much distress and, because every family's problems differ, general 'rules' will not always apply.

However, lawyers agree that many problems will be avoided if a brain-impaired person has died leaving a will. This means, in fact, that everybody should make a will before it is too late. Certainly, no one should wait until the winter of his life before bequeathing property. Those diagnosed as having dementia may still be able to sign legal documents, although, as one Australian lawyer points out, they are wide open to being duped and relatives should come to an arrangement where a qualified member of the legal profession is present during the drawing up and signing of the will.

Day-to-day affairs will still need to be managed, and if a dementing person is incapable of signing papers, a trusted relative should be in possession of a letter, warrant or power of attorney that gives him or her the legal right to sign documents on behalf of the afflicted person. Of course, the person still has to sign a document in the first place handing over that authority, so again the position arises of needing to have everything properly signed up before it is too late.

And if it is too late? If a person has gone beyond the point of 'reason'? Relatives might then find themselves involved in a court case to contest a will or to seek the acquisition of property. Under Australia's Family Law Act, 1975, the Alzheimer sufferer would be represented by a guardian — someone who acts to protect the rights of that person in the proceedings. The Attorney-General may, for example, appoint the Public Trustee of the State to act on behalf of the person. Usually, it is not the guardian who starts legal proceedings.

When a family challenges a will, the Probate Court will require evidence about the testamentary capacity of the afflicted person. A lawyer applying for probate will have to prove that if someone who died from an Alzheimer type disease had made a will, he was capable of knowing what he was doing when he made it. Complicated legal questions will also arise if the person had been suffering from mental problems brought on by the following:

Depression A person suffering from this may have feelings of guilt that he and his family have committed sins and they are not worthy of a share in his estate. There have been cases where the assets of the estate have been given to charity and the family left with nothing.

Cerebro-vascular disease This can cause a fluctuation in a person's mental state which may not mean that he is incapable of making a will. The lawyer involved will have to be satisfied, along with witnesses, that the testator is in a clear state of mind. If there is any doubt, a doctor should be asked to give a certificate stating the testamentary capacity.

Paranoia A family may be cut out of a will if a sufferer believes that a husband or wife has been unfaithful. A lawyer would be required in court to prove that the testator was suffering from this problem.

Alcoholism A court might find that a person suffering from this was incapable of signing a will, particularly if he has displayed antagonism against his family.

Sexual behaviour

The end of 'normal' functioning of the brain does not mean the death of a sexual relationship. Many people at the onset of dementia still desire sexual contact and are capable of enjoying it. At the same time, some might behave undesirably in public, exposing themselves or rubbing their genitals. Obviously, this is not done to deliberately upset those around. It feels good, and the person is not aware of the reactions of others. You can expect all types of behaviour — mischievous, amusing, downright outrageous. The confused brain causes the person to act in many different ways, and some families have been stunned by their relative's behaviour.

Sons report mothers trying to seduce them, fathers expose themselves to their daughters, women fondle their breasts in restaurants, men make suggestions to shoppers in the supermarket. Such anti-social behaviour will shock, and the best thing to do is to lead your relative away to a quiet private area and try to distract him by talking to him or giving him something else to do.

Such behaviour does not affect everyone. Sometimes if people take their clothes off and sit around the house naked or walk down the street with nothing on, there is no sexual urge behind these actions.

Often they are hot, uncomfortable or simply forgetful. If there is a sexual urge, it is probably because the person is looking for physical comfort or some form of assurance. In one Sydney nursing home, for example, to the amusement of the night staff, two old ladies were constantly disrobing and clambering into bed together.

Sometimes you can help quell a sexual urge by grasping the person's hand or stroking the face or arm. If your relative wants love, give it in the best way *you* feel capable of. Certainly the worst way of dealing with sexual desire or antisocial behaviour is to be angry with your relative and tell him what a dirty person he is. He is reacting to an inner feeling. To strike at such natural instincts with harsh words only adds to the confusion and frustration.

Hallucinations and delusions

There may be times when your dementing relative talks about things that are not there in reality. He might smell fire, think his clothes are wet, say his food is cold when it's hot. He will accuse you of taking something belonging to him, think that somebody is 'after' him. He may pluck at the air.

When people are hallucinating, they see things that no one else can. When they believe things that are not a fact, they are suffering from delusion. Often, a dementing person moves between hallucination and delusion. Wives might say their partners are not their husbands — that they are strangers who do not belong in their bed. Husbands might say that the house they are in is not their real home. Without causing an argument, you might reply that you are the person who married him or her in 19-- and that this is where you have both lived for years. Remind your relative of your children or sisters or brothers; it might give him some assurance that you really are part of the family. Failure to recognise people, a condition known as agnosia, is something you will come to expect as your relative's disease progresses.

Families have found that the best way of tackling wrong impressions is not to disagree but to reach a compromise so that the carer is not put into a position where he or she has to admit a mistake and the Alzheimer victim has the last word. To constantly agree with the sufferer when you know he is wrong and you are right only lessens your own self-esteem and can take away an edge of your confidence.

Mobility

Invariably, dementia sufferers experience problems with movement. A tiny crack in the pavement, for instance, can look to them like a wide chasm. And the pavement edge, a big drop. Sufferers are afraid to step out because it means taking one foot off the ground and they might fall. Their sense of balance is diminished; they lose the confidence to stand unassisted and therefore grasp at objects and people.

When an Alzheimer sufferer starts walking with small steps, he is displaying symptoms similar to those affected by Parkinson's disease. Both conditions, in fact, arise from a similar type of brain impairment. Dyspraxia — difficulty in organising movement — is a problem for some people, while in others there may be problems with postural righting reflexes. These righting reflexes automatically set in chain movements to correct any tendency to fall over, but when impaired a person seems frail and tottery and can literally trip over a bus ticket.

When your relative reaches the stage of the *marche a petits pas*, you will have to be at his side. Offer him your arm to grasp. Sometimes the grip will be unbearably tight. A London woman has made herself a wide 'bracelet' of foam rubber to relieve the pressure of her husband's grasp when she leads him around the house.

Should your relative fall, he might be able to help himself up to a great extent — it is natural for any human or animal to try to get back up after a tumble. To help your fallen relative after you have checked he has not injured himself, manoeuvre him into a kneeling position. Then encourage him to put one foot forward on which he can push himself up with your assistance. You must take care that you do not strain yourself while bringing a person to his feet. Don't lean forward, bending your back, when you lift because you could damage your spine. Keep your back straight, and bend at the knees. Don't grasp your relative by the hands and attempt to pull him forwards and up — if he's frail, you could wrench bones from their sockets. If you can get him into a sitting position, reach in under his armpits from behind, locking hands across the chest. Have your weight firmly distributed so you are well balanced, and lift so that the strain is taken by your thighs. You must use your legs, not your back. Demented people are like a dead weight. Lifting them can sometimes be too much for one person, and a neighbour's help should be sought if you feel any strain. If there's a chair handy, bring it to the fallen person — he may be able to use it for support when trying to stand.

Physiotherapy

Staff at Melbourne's Royal Southern Memorial Hospital and associated physiotherapists working with the elderly have drawn up guidelines to assist carers in physical management — and assist the elderly themselves to maintain their independence wherever possible.

Like colleagues around the world, they emphasise that if you know that a person can manage a task alone, do not help, but stand by if necessary to give confidence and encouragement. Even people with dementing illnesses can undertake many tasks, and you should encourage them to remain independent as long as possible. The following suggestions will help both you and your dementing relative.

Standing up from a chair or bed First, the person should be asked to push himself to the edge of the chair or sit on the edge of the bed. Next, ask him to tuck his feet under the edge of the bed or chair so that his 'nose is over his toes'. Then, with his hands on the arms of the chair or on the seat or the bed, ask him to push up with his hands and knees. Even if he requires assistance, this procedure should be followed. The person should then be standing, but it is a good idea to ask him to stand still for about ten seconds before commencing moving. Elderly people should be encouraged to sit in a chair that is not too low, so they do not experience difficulty when standing up.

Walking If walking aids are required, they should always be used, rather than allowing a person to rely on someone else for help. Of course, care should be taken when four-point sticks or walking frames are used on uneven ground to ensure that all four legs are on the same level. Should a person want to turn a corner, remind him to step around the corner and not pivot on one foot.

Moving from chair to chair When transferring a person from one chair to another, it is best to have the chairs either facing one another or at right angles to each other. If transferring to or from a wheelchair, make sure the brakes are on and the footplates up. Should the person be able to do these things himself, encourage him to do them. Having got him to his feet (as explained in 'Standing up from a chair or bed'), help the person on his weaker side and ask him to place his stronger arm on the opposite arm of the chair to be sat on. He should now turn so that his bottom is over the seat of the chair, and the edge of the seat can be felt at the backs of his legs. With his hands on the arms of the chair, he should lower himself gently — never flop.

Walking up and down stairs When using steps or stairs, encourage a person to use the handrail, if there is one. Assistance can be given by supporting under the arm on the side away from the handrail. A four-point stick or walking frame can be carried to the top or bottom of the stairs before walking up or down. If assistance is not necessary, walk ahead when going down stairs and behind when going up stairs. If a person has one leg stronger than the other, that leg should be used first when going up stairs and last when going down stairs. As a visiting priest once commented, to help people remember which leg to use first: 'Good leg to heaven, bad leg to hell!'

Exercise It is very important that an elderly person does not sit too long in the same position. Long periods of immobility are very debilitating; an hour in the same position is long enough. If possible, the elderly person should be encouraged to take a short walk at least once an hour.

While sitting, the following simple exercises can be performed, which will help maintain tone in the muscles required for walking:
1. Straighten each knee alternately, six times.
2. Bend and stretch both ankles, six times.
3. Tighten the tummy muscles and squeeze the buttocks together, six times.
4. Push up on the arm of the chair and ease the buttocks off the seat of the chair, four times.

Easing pain A hot water bottle can help aching joints, but care should be taken to ensure that it is well wrapped so that burning does not occur. The wrapping can be gradually removed as the bottle cools. Moist heat is particularly beneficial for back pain or arthritic joints.

Baths and showers These are excellent for aching muscles and joints. And stiff painful fingers and wrists can be exercised while immersed in a basin of warm water.

Ice packs Some people get more relief from the application of ice rather than heat. An ice pack can be made by wrapping several

crushed ice cubes in two or three layers of damp towel. It should
then be applied to the painful joints or muscles for ten minutes.

Foot care

The care of feet is an essential but often-neglected area. Here are
guidelines for the elderly who do not have any significant problems
with their feet. Daily care is very important.
1. Keep the feet clean. If the person is unable to get into a bath, feet
should be soaked daily in warm water and weak detergent. Pat dry
with a soft towel and do not use talcum powder between the toes.
2. If circulation is poor, make sure the patient's extremities are
kept very warm. Slacks or trousers will keep legs warm, and wool-
len socks will help to prevent chilblains. The person must not sit
too close to fires and heaters and should not leave feet on a hot
water bottle for lengthy periods.
3. Use of an emollient cream each day is advisable, as with age the
skin becomes dry. Lesion breakdown is less likely if the skin is kept
elastic.
4. Wear comfortable shoes. At home, do not wear slippers in day
time. If the aged foot has deformities, shoes must accommodate
these rather than further cramp them. Shoes with thicker soles are
more comfortable. As part of the ageing process, we lose our adi-
pose, or fatty tissue, and shoes with very thin soles can be painful.
5. Adhesive pads should not be used on an elderly person's foot
because the hard layers of skin can soften and become susceptible
to infection. Sponge insoles are the correct choice.
6. If the person has arthritis or conditions that make the weight of
bedclothes painful, a cradle can be placed in the bed and the clothes
arranged around it.
7. Older people should rest their feet for about an hour a day,
either on the bed or with the legs elevated. Shoes should be removed.

Teeth

If you do not keep a dementing person's mouth clean and the teeth
in good order, you will find that problems increase. Not only is his
health likely to suffer, but his impairment will worsen, for poor

oral hygiene can poison the whole system. Yet along with the feet, teeth and gums are the most neglected areas of the human body.

In the early stages of dementia, while visits to the dentist are still easy to arrange, make sure that your relative sees the dentist every six months. If the mouth remains in good health, you will avoid trauma later on. As his mental decline continues, switch to yearly visits, but carry on with your daily oral hygiene programme. If your relative objects, try to choose a time of the day when you know he is in a calmer frame of mind. A good place to check his mouth and clean his teeth is in the bath.

Don't assume that because your relative is capable of still caring for himself that he is not neglecting his mouth — it might be the area he continually forgets. Dentures, for instance, can be irritating if they don't fit well or if the denture adhesive is not properly applied. Leave the person to do as much for himself as possible, but be aware that he may need direction, as teeth cleaning is fiddly.

Nutrition

Diet is of vital importance. Poor nutrition might not be a contributing factor to dementia, but it certainly doesn't help in the fight against it. What hope does the human body have against a constant onslaught by junk food, chemical additives, lashings of salt and sugar, high fat contents, frozen TV dinners, overboiled vegetables, sweets and refined breads? We all need nutrition, and our bodies have to search rather hard for it among the highly refined soft foods so often consumed. In those suffering from dementia, the immune system is already fighting hard against chemical changes in the brain and which ultimately work their way through the whole system. Good nutrition helps to build the body's defences, and any advice that suggests no special nutritional requirements are needed for a dementing person should be ignored. We all need foods rich in vitamins and minerals.

It's easy to suggest change, but not so easy to implement it when people have spent a lifetime eating a certain way. It is difficult to feed someone steamed fish when he has been used to eating fried fish in thick batter all his life, accompanied by a pile of salty chips. Many will stubbornly refuse any new foods in the diet, so changes have to be introduced gradually. A sudden and radical change in food will probably bring about a strong refusal, yet the changes don't have to be radical. For instance, if you are relying on white refined breads for both yourself and your relative, what about substituting these with their wholegrain counterparts — wholegrain bread instead of white; brown rice instead of white; wholemeal pasta instead of white pasta (even egg noodles are better than the flour-and-water type). And, instead of peeling and scraping your vegetables, eat them with the skins on.

If the person accepts this 'new' way of eating, don't give him a 'treat' of fried food one day, because you'll more than likely have to start the process all over again. Of course, if a change of food fails, it will be necessary to supplement the diet with vitamin tablets. Older people tend to suffer a zinc deficiency, which has been suggested as a contributing factor in dementia. But if you are going to give a person suffering from dementia mineral and vitamin supplements, check with your doctor about quantity.

Dementing people tend to have difficulty at meal times. They are often confused when using knives and forks, and in time you might have to cut their food up for them and give them a spoon. Eventually, even the ability to use the spoon might be lost and you will have to help them. But encourage them to participate in meal times and feed themselves for as long as possible. In severe cases, make sure the person has a napkin on his lap and is wearing a bib. Sometimes the afflicted person will reach out with his hand for food on your plate, so beware of that. If he insists on eating his food with his fingers, it might be easier in the long run to allow him to continue to do so. At all costs, you must ensure that your relative eats and drinks enough, because when dementing people stop eating or if they become dehydrated there is a danger they will develop bacterial or viral pneumonia.

If you cannot get your relative to eat, try a liquid diet — vegetable juices and other liquidised solids. Don't force him to eat a second meal in the day if he doesn't want one. And if he indicates he wants food after having just had a meal, it's not necessarily because he is still hungry — he's simply forgotten he has eaten.

Some sufferers have 'dyspraxic' difficulties with swallowing. They may chew endlessly but have trouble actually initiating the complex act of swallowing. They may need to be reminded or asked to swallow. Sometimes they might spit food out. Try putting less on the spoon if you are feeding your relative and wait for him to chew it. As always, patience is the key, so try to ensure that meal times are without stress.

It should be remembered that when activity levels fall, foods of poor nutritional value — for example, refined carbohydrates and alcohol — should be reduced. And foods rich in vitamins and minerals — vitamin C, calcium, folate, iron and fibre — should be increased. It is not a bad idea to include lecithin, too. Although controlled medical tests suggest that soya bean extract does not help, some families have found that including it in a dementing person's diet over a long period of time has improved alertness. Another suggestion is to break down meals into six smaller portions instead of three larger ones.

Feed your relative and yourself live fresh foods: constipation of the body results in constipation of the mind. Don't think that roughage means only bran, bran, bran. Include in your diet whole grains, fibrous lightly cooked vegetables and salads, and fruit. Remember that green leafy vegetables are rich in chlorophyll and not only clean out a sluggish system but also diminish body odour.

Daily food guide for adults

Group 1 — milk and milk products This group contains milk, yellow cheese, white cheese (cottage and ricotta), yoghurt, ice cream and buttermilk. Milk is a major supplier of calcium, needed for building bones and teeth, fighting blood clotting, sound heartbeat, healthy nervous system. From this group you also get protein, needed for growth and repair of body tissues. Each day you need at least 300 mL of milk. One cup (250 mL or 8 oz) is equal to 30 g (1 oz) of yellow cheese: 250 g (8 oz) of white cheese; 200 g (7 oz) of yoghurt; five scoops of ice cream.

Group 2 — meat and meat equivalents This group contains meat, fish, poultry, eggs, nuts, pulses (lentils, dried peas and beans) and seeds (sesame seeds, and so on). This group is a major supplier of protein, iron and B vitamins. Protein, of course, is needed for the growth and repair of body tissues; iron is essential for a healthy blood supply; and the B vitamins are for energy use, a healthy digestive tract and healthy skin. You need at least one serving from this group (90 g or 3 oz per serving). 90 g of meat is equal to three eggs, one cup of cooked pulses or 90 g of nuts or seeds.

Group 3 — fruit and vegetables This group includes citrus fruits such as oranges, lemons, grapefruit, and alternatives such as tomatoes and pineapples; dark green leafy vegetables, such as silverbeet, spinach, broccoli, brussels sprouts; yellow vegetables, such as pumpkin and carrot; other fruits and vegetables, including potato. In this group are found vitamin C, needed for growth and maintenance of strong gums and all other tissues and the healing of wounds; fibre, for a healthy digestive tract; carbohydrate, for energy; vitamin A, for eyesight and skin; and iron, for blood supply. Daily you need four or more servings from this group including one of citrus, one of dark green leafy vegetables, one of yellow vegetables, and two of other fruit and vegetables.

Group 4 — bread and cereals Contained in this group are bread; breakfast cereals; pastas; rice. These are major suppliers of carbohydrate for energy; B vitamins for energy use; fibre for a healthy digestive tract; and iron for blood supply. You need four or more servings from this group each day, one serving equalling a slice of bread or half a cup of cooked cereal or pasta. Wholegrains are important.

Group 5 — fats and oils This group contains butter, margarine, oil, salad dressings and cream. These products are major suppliers of fat, needed for concentrated energy; vitamin A for healthy eyes and skin; and vitamin D for strong bones and teeth. You need 15 to 30g a day (1/2–1 oz or 1–2 tablespoons).

Nutrition-related disease commonly found in the elderly

1. Obesity. Develops when the energy intake is greater than energy expenditure.
2. Coronary heart disease. May be due to excessive intake of cholesterol and saturated fats, refined carbohydrate and/or alcohol.
3. Diabetes mellitus (especially maturity onset diabetes). More prevalent among people suffering from obesity.
4. Diverticulosis. Inadequate fibre (roughage) in diet.
5. Simple constipation. Inadequate fibre.
6. Cancer of the large bowel. Inadequate fibre in diet, longer transit time of faecal material, increased exposure of carcinogenic substances to the bowel wall.
7. Iron deficiency anaemia. Inadequate dietary intake of iron.

Emergency stores

Carers looking after dementing people, or those in the early stages
of dementia who are still able to manage on their own, or elderly
people living alone, should all ensure there is an adequate stock of
food items for weekends or emergency situations. Such emergencies can arise through illness, transport difficulties, financial difficulties or poor weather. The supplies should be non-perishable,
have a shelf-life of at least two weeks, not require much cooking or
preparation and have some nutritional value. Here is a suggested
grocery cupboard for those emergency situations:

Cheese: round cartons with individually wrapped portions to avoid
drying out or mould.

Evaporated milk; and powdered or instant milk.

Canned fish: tuna, salmon, sardines.

Canned or dried stews and soups containing meat and vegetables.

Dried apricots, prunes, sultanas, dates.

Canned fruit and juices, especially citrus and tomato.

Bread, preferably wholegrain: rye is best of all; and the packaged
(imported) varieties such as pumpernickel will keep well on the
shelf; refrigerate after opening.

Frozen vegetables: sprouts, broccoli, peas, carrots.

Canned salad vegetables: asparagus, beetroot, beans, peas, potato
salad, tomato.

Packets of crispbreads: Ryvita and Nutravite.

Breakfast cereals: muesli, oatmeal (porridge), bran, wholegrain bis-
cuits.

Tea, coffee, cocoa, Aktavite.

Fresh fruit for weekends.

Milk-based instant desserts; custard powder; junket tablets.

The big dilemma: home care or institution?

Whatever doctors suggest, whatever friends and neighbours feel, it
is the immediate family of an Alzheimer sufferer, those who have to
deal with the day-to-day problems, who are the only people in a
position to make the ultimate decision: to keep the afflicted person
at home or send him away to a nursing home.

   Such decisions are not faced at the onset of dementia. The

afflicted person acts oddly compared with previous behaviour, but in the early stages his family are usually not convinced that his actions warrant handing him over to the care of strangers, particularly if he is a loved and respected member of the family. In most cases, families decide to 'give it a go'. They do not see their relative as being so badly impaired that he cannot continue to be incorporated into the family circle. They believe they can offer greater security and comfort at home, and there is the general impression that nursing homes and institutions are 'the end of the line'. While a family member remains at home, there is still hope.

These are the usual considerations at the beginning, after dementia has been diagnosed. In addition, specialists will encourage families to keep their relatives at home because of the pressure on nursing home beds. And there are financial considerations, too. Keeping a person in a good nursing home is not cheap, despite government relief, and families believe they can give better care, more cheaply, by keeping their relative at home.

At first, families cope reasonably well, researchers have found. They explain their relative's 'peculiar' behaviour to neighbours and friends; they learn to live with the forgetfulness, the repetitive questions, the moods, the wanderings. If the burden is shared by family members operating a rota system, relatives are able to go about their own day-to-day activities almost as before.

If the task of caring falls upon one person, most activities have to stop, but life is not bad enough to — as many would see it — 'push' their relative into a home. However, families have found that life does not get easier as the dementia progresses. Even if the march of the disease can be halted, whatever damage has been done will usually remain. There is a belief among some medical researchers that areas of the brain can be trained to take on the tasks that the dead areas once performed. Of course, everyone is different, and it is natural for relatives to always hold out some hope. Sometimes the decision to keep a person at home defies all logic.

An 89-year-old Sydney man could not be left alone because he often wandered on to a busy road. His daughter-in-law, a clinical laboratory supervisor, decided to give up her job to care for him. In essence, it seemed a good solution. But the family lost her income, the government lost a significant amount of income tax, society lost her skilled productivity, and she gave up a 40-hour-a-week job for a 168-hour-a-week responsibility. As one doctor who knows the woman commented: 'Such a solution may have been valid when the demand upon a woman's labour was unlimited and its value trivial because she was not considered to be in the work force. Today, women's skills are valuable and such a "solution" does not make much sense. In addition, it can be argued that it is not cost effective and that the resultant isolation of the father-in-law from his aged peers might actually reduce the amount of social interaction, activity and stimulation.'

Families who take on the responsibility of care open the door to a great many personal problems. Generally, when Alzheimer's disease or a related disorder has been diagnosed, the person is going to become progressively more difficult to manage. His decline might be rapid — particularly if the disease is diagnosed at an early age such as the forties or fifties — or take many years before a 'living corpse' condition is reached. When the changes are rapid, the frustration and difficulties for the carer are magnified. Within a year or two, the overworked family member might find himself or herself dealing with urinary and faecal incontinence — often the factor that forces decisions about homes to be reached. But it's a terrible scenario to face: a relative, perhaps in his fifties, being placed in a nursing home. When the disease creeps into the brain of an older person, its progress is usually more gradual, so that nursing home considerations do not arise until later years.

Problems can arise almost from the beginning where families are not united or when there is no younger person at hand to share the burden of care. If the wife of a frail elderly husband becomes a victim of mental impairment, it would be beyond his capabilities to look after her. Probably the best solution would be for her to go to a home, and there would be a strong argument for him to be placed there with her in a private room so that neither is left to cope with strangers and loneliness.

One of the paradoxes of medical science is that in lengthening life expectancy it has created difficulties for those inheriting those extra years — and for their relatives. A couple of centuries ago, people were dying in their fifties and sixties, and although they were cared for at home their 'children' were younger than the adult children of today, whose parents are into their seventies and eighties. The longer we live, the greater the chances of developing some form of dementia or other illness. Many ailments can be successfully treated, of course, but irreversible dementia has to be *managed*.

And if that management is beyond the scope or tolerance of individuals and families, the question of nursing home placement looms. It is always a painful decision. Some families say they feel guilty even considering a home for the person who was once as normal as the rest of them. Sometimes they see flashes of the 'old' personality and they wonder whether their dementing relative is aware that a decision is about to be made about them. This only adds to the carer's frustration.

But the time will come when social life becomes extremely restricted, friends drop away, and the carer feels physically and mentally worn out. The carer loses sleep because of the afflicted person's night cries or wanderings or bed wetting. It becomes a traumatic experience to dash to the shops because anything could happen while the carer is away, and the home is filled with tension. There is no outside stimulation, no conversation, no shared enjoyment of a television show — nothing but cooking, mopping up, wiping, watching, changing, cleaning. Some people can cope with all this; many, after years of it, say 'Enough!'.

When, after struggling on to the point of exhaustion, the carer decides that an institution should be considered, two factors loom: cost and guilt. Most western governments provide some form of financial relief for families who have no alternative but to seek out a nursing home. Of course, the type of aid varies from country to country, from government to government. Nursing home care does not come cheap. In Australia, for example, Mrs Betts has put her mother in a home which charges $446.60 a week. The government subsidises the cost with a contribution of $341.60, leaving Mrs Betts to find $105. 'It's like I'm buying freedom,' she says. 'I'm sure most people would happily pay $105 a week not to be confined in a prison. Of course, I still make my visits, which can cut into the day, but it's not like being trapped in the house. I don't feel any guilt about having my mother where she is — I felt I wasn't able to care for her as well as I was able at the beginning. I just became tired out.' As Mrs Betts says, she feels no guilt about placing her mother in a home. Even though her mother is not getting personal attention, she is able to walk around, is being fed regularly and is in the company of others, which might give her some daily stimulation.

Before taking the final decision, a family conference is advisable to discuss the whole situation. Sometimes carers have found that some of their family members will make criticisms, saying how wrong it is to even consider a nursing home, yet these are often the people who have given little home support, who have never experienced the day-to-day problems at first hand. If you are the carer, the final decision should rest with you if there is any family dissent.

So you decide on nursing home placement. But that is not the end of your problems. The next hurdle is *finding* a home with a vacant bed. As one state government community worker in Australia says: 'Families think they can make a decision and have mum or dad in a home by the end of the week. It's not that easy. There is a huge demand on beds, and quite often you just have to take what you can when you can. Most times, it's a case of take it or leave it. Some homes are quite terrible.'

One Melbourne woman, in a letter to her Member of Parliament in March 1984, complained there were substantially more than 1000 demented patients throughout Victoria with nowhere to go because the government had 'deliberately withheld' the granting of licences for the opening of new nursing homes. 'These unfortunate aged and infirmed citizens who need special nursing care are therefore being deprived of this service,' she wrote.

The woman, whose mother is dementing, had many more strong words to say. 'The government is creating chaos and heartache for so many families by forcing them to look after nursing home cases at home. These patients are really beyond the scope of unqualified home nursing, some being incontinent, others confused, or both, and who are receiving minimal amounts of practical aid from the nursing service and local government in the form of home help, Meals on Wheels and so on ...

'I suggest that MPs should each take a stroll around a well-organised nursing home, and you will realise that the average citizen is not trained to cope with these confused patients. It all requires a specialised, devoted nursing talent, which we do not all magically possess. Also, the nursing staff can move away from the situation at the end of their shift, whereas the family is compelled to go on caring and tending to the patient continually in the home situation 24 hours a day.'

She concluded: 'The whole situation is a disastrous mess, and you must consider altering the situation very promptly or our whole medical system will be in chaos.'

The same problem exists in many other countries as the number of mentally impaired people grows. Homes are bursting at the seams, and there are long waiting lists. What makes it particularly difficult for families is that many homes say they will not take Alzheimer patients because they are unpredictable and uncontrollable. One group of social workers in Melbourne suggests a 'bed rota system' so that patients spend time in a nursing home and time with their relatives. This breaks down the problem of one group of people being permanently in an institution, another permanently at home.

Having made your decision to seek out a bed, you can only wait and hope. If, as can sometimes happen, you suddenly have a choice of two or three homes, a personal inspection is a must. Do the staff strike you as friendly and caring? Does the home use restraints? If so, you might feel this practice will cause too much frustration for your relative. Can you visit at hours convenient to you? Is there a pleasant outdoor setting? The food, what is it like — nutritious or prepared from frozen vegetables or overcooked?

Try to envisage your relative going to a second home — a place that provides close to everything you were able to give in your own house. You won't be able to find an exact replica, but you might come close to it. And look for 'hidden' extras such as the cost of medicines, incontinence pads, laundry charges, and so on. There are good homes and bad homes, and it is often difficult to make an assessment on a first visit. Some observations made by welfare groups are favourable, but others can be horrifying. In Australia, the Lithuanian Women's Welfare Organisation said in a report: 'Existing private institutions are brutal and inhumane. We know of one case where an elderly brain-damaged Lithuanian eats tea leaves. We take food to supplement the diet he is given.'

For migrants entering a home, there can be problems. Removed from the family environment, away from relatives who speak their language, they withdraw. Joan Keane, a Melbourne social worker reports: 'When psychiatric disturbance or dementia makes them unmanageable in the family, they have to be placed in nursing or rest homes. In a strange environment, away from all that is familiar and dear to them, they have nothing to do but sit and wait for death.'

Yet a New South Wales woman writes of a nursing home-rehabilitation centre, where her mother was staying: 'When she arrived in this rehabilitation centre my mother was almost done for. Angry, very depressed, in pain from a broken hip, and totally confused by the changes in her life. And now this environment is working miracles on her. Sometimes she is content just to sit and gaze at the surroundings. There is a lot of greenery and shapes of the plants in their variety. I brush my mother's silky-white handful of hair and remember that she told me she used to brush her mother's hair. She tilts her face back, and I massage it with oily face cream, feeling the bones under her spare flesh, soft, female skin. We are both enjoying it ... and I, with my usual greed, want to hold this moment, want to banish the anger and sadness and panic that will come again ...'

Some 80 out of 100 men and 90 out of 100 women in nursing homes have no wives or husbands, suggesting that age and disability are manageable as long as there is a competent companion. About 19 per cent of those in nursing homes have never been married. When childless marriages and family separations are added, there will be even more people with no children to provide an alternative home. One solution showing promise is the personal-care home, or special accommodation house, in which a family undertakes to care for several residents. Although this method has been used for psychiatric patients, its potential for geriatric patients has not been equally well explored. At present, the costs are reasonable, but it is possible that with improvement of standards, these costs would also rise.

Dr Cees van Tiggelen, the Dutch psychogeriatrician working in Australia, contends that nursing homes, hostels and similar establishments should not necessarily be the end of the line for elderly people, even though this seems to be the general belief among would-be residents and their relatives. 'Through proper management, most elderly will still be able to enjoy life. The management, philosophy and even design of such places can contribute to allowing their elderly guests getting the most out of life,' he says.

His views are supported by Brian Moss, Director of Melbourne's Moorfields Community for Adult Care, who has just prepared a lengthy report on care of the aged around the world. 'A nursing home should be a place to live, not a place to die,' he says. Criticising the lack of adequate assessement services for people appearing to be suffering from senile dementia, Moss comments: 'Too often, elderly people are assumed to be afflicted because of behaviour patterns, or because they are old. Appropriate assessment procedures would show whether the condition is due to pseudodementia or reversible dementia, both of which can be treated. Unfortunately, we sentence many elderly people to a lifetime in nursing homes or other institutions where the problem is often compounded by the injudicious use of drugs.'

If it is at all possible, then, you should shop around. Dr van Tiggelen's expectations of what a home should offer may help you to make a decision.

What is important, he says, is the layout of the building. It is not always practical or possible, but the design should encourage physical activity. It is far better to have a couple of toilets in the corridor than attached to bedrooms. People have to walk to them. For psychogeriatric patients, a square or rectangular building with corridors in each wing will enable a patient to walk around without coming to a closed door.

Wards have to be personal. Small group or individual nursing is a good idea in a geriatric ward. A big ward with 30 or so people gets impersonal. At van Tiggelen's hospital, a bedroom was converted to a living room to accommodate ten people. Wards of 30 patients were rearranged into units for ten. The units had their own dining rooms, and the residents ate in smaller groups, instead of in a cafeteria atmosphere. Each unit had its own nurses who didn't wear uniforms, so each group of patients and staff lived together.

In any home away from home, residents must feel welcome. This starts from the moment they enter the hostel, nursing home or hospital. Too often, a patient is admitted on an hour's notice and all that is known about him is what drugs he is on. But if staff already know his background, something of his likes and dislikes and his family, he will feel more welcome and keep his identity.

Part of this feeling of being at home comes from having familiar things around. A person might like their favourite pictures or a crucifix to hang on the wall, their own cup and saucer, or bedspread, chair, clock, newspaper. Van Tiggelen recalls a mentally disturbed old lady being admitted to his hospital. She had lived on a farm and always wore an apron, except on Sundays. When she was admitted, her daughter was too embarrassed to take in her old aprons and bought her new dresses. The old lady became more and more distressed and cried a lot. Then she started tearing her clothes, crying 'I have to milk the cows'. An imaginative nurse connected the clothes with the old lady's distress and asked her daughter to bring in her old clothes. The old lady put them on and did not cry out again. She was, says the doctor, cured.

In an institution, nutrition is an essential part of keeping people healthy; but this does not mean that meals have to be dull. As well, meal times can play a vital part in people keeping their dignity.

Placement is important. If some patients do not get on, staff have to ensure they are not seated near each other. People usually raise or lower themselves to their surroundings. If a meal is set out with tables decorated and decent crockery is used, the residents will, on the whole, adjust to this environment. If people are given plastic plates and plastic cutlery, they will probably grab their food with their hands.

Preparation of food is usually a lifetime occupation of women. As 60 to 70 per cent of those in institutions are women who have spent decades preparing food, why should they be denied a basic right to continue that occupation when admitted to an institution? The cook would probably not approve of patients helping in the kitchen, but there should be provisions when building a nursing home for a small area where patients can bake scones if they wish.

Physical and occupational therapy is often presented in a negative way. Unless it has some fun element, an old person usually doesn't see the point in it — particularly someone with communication disorders. Dancing is always enjoyed by the elderly, and waltzes should be played in the recreation room. Animals can be far more therapeutic than bottles of medication. A cat, a dog or a cockatoo around a nursing home gives many elderly people something to take a keen interest in.

Rules and regulations, van Tiggelen suggests, should be abolished in nursing homes. Patients shold be left to choose whether they want a meal or not, whether they want to go to bed, or whether they want to make tea for their visitors. Obviously for those unable to decide for themselves about eating, they should be led to the dining table at the appropriate time.

'Nursing homes', says van Tiggelen, 'should cultivate an environment where people should be able to live to the full extent. Nursing home care too often is directed towards looking after a person's handicaps and not encouraging his strengths. Far too often, nursing homes, particularly those built on hospital grounds, are managed according to hospital lines, which does not encourage individuality. These attitudes stem from the top. There's a big difference in patients in a hostel or nursing home with an active, stimulating supervisor and one run by an old-fashioned authoritarian matron who decides everything. In the first case, people are encouraged into all sorts of activities, so when new patients are admitted, they happily join in. That is the pressure of the peer group. In the second case, you may go into the sitting room where all the patients are kept quiet, lined up along the walls in front of a switched-off television set. New patients join in, too.'

Government benefits for carers at home

For those who are able to care for their afflicted relative at home, temporary relief from pressures can be found. Big cities have some form of home help facilities where a nurse calls to bathe the dementing person so the relative can at least go to the hairdresser or the shops. In cases where it is essential for carers to continue their work, they can get relief by having their relative attend a day centre or day hospital. Attendance varies from one to five days a week, and transport is usually available. Some charges are involved, and as these vary you should make enquiries about what is available at what cost in your area. Home nurses are also available to give the person a walk or bath.

In Australia, if you have a nurse calling, you are entitled to Domiciliary Care Benefits paid by the federal government. Some hospitals will take your relative for a week or so while you take a holiday, but as soon as you admit them, you lose the domiciliary care benefit temporarily. You'll lose it, too, if you take your relative away with you for a week or more. What this means, in fact, is that the system of paying the relative a small amount for the care he or she is giving, ties the carer to the house. Special benefits of about $80 a week are also available to those who give up their work or careers to care for their incapacitated relative, but this means that all initiative is destroyed. A carer who wants to continue to use his or her intellect to further a career from home is not, under the rules of special benefit payments, allowed to do anything else but devote all his or her time to household duties.

A Sydney daughter: 'I wanted to continue running my dressmaking business from the house. I could cope with looking after my father and my elderly mother while working at the sewing machine, but when the government inspector from the Social Services Department found out, he told me I couldn't conduct a business while receiving special benefits or they would take money from me. I needed the government money to help because the business wouldn't have made much. So I had to give up all hope of working from home. Instead, I turned into a kind of moron, caring, caring, caring, with only a pittance from the government. And I had to declare it as income to the tax man! The government really ought to give people like me some incentive, not beat us down to domestic slaves.'

A West Australian woman: 'By keeping my sister at home, I'm saving the government $20 000 a year, which is what it costs to keep her in a nursing home. Surely, instead of paralysing people, they should give us some tax incentive. I would rather work at home and get a tax break than get a pension and become a vegetable and end up in a home as well, suffering from a dead mind — and then, at the going rate of inflation, it would cost the government $30 000.'

The Australian Department of Social Security explains it this way: 'On Special Benefits, you can get the same amount of money as you receive on unemployment benefit. However, there are variations according to a family's circumstances. If you earn $20 a week, your benefit payment of $73.60 is not affected. But income of $20 to $70 means that the Special Benefits are reduced by 50 cents in the dollar. If you earn between $70 and $118 a week, you lose dollar for dollar. In simple terms, your benefit payment is cancelled out if you earn a figure which is greater than the payment.' (These figures are subject to change.)

Some facts and figures to guide Australian residents, who need to do some sums to assess home care, are:

Age pension This is payable to all men aged 65 or older and all women aged 60 or older who are permanent residents and have lived in Australia for a minimum of two years. The payment rate is increased twice yearly in May and November with the cost-of-living adjustments. Current pension rates are: Single pension $85.90, reduced when income exceeds $30; pension cuts out when income reaches $201.80. Married pension $143.20 (combined payment), reduced when income exceeds $50; pension cuts out when income reaches $336.40.

Over-70 pension rates Those over 70 are eligible for the same maximum rate of pension as other current rates, but a more generous means test applies: Single pension $51.45 when income is $98.90 to $200; pension cuts out when income is $302.90. Married pension $85.80 (combined payment) when income is $164.80 to $333; pension cuts out when income is $504.60.

Spouse carer's pension This has been introduced for men who have to give constant care and attention to their wives, who are severely handicapped by a physical or intellectual disability and are living at home. To qualify for the pension, wives must be paid age pension, invalid pension or rehabilitation allowance (providing she was eligible for invalid pension immediately prior to rehabilitation allowance being granted). A spouse carer's pension cannot be paid at the same time as any other pension or benefit or rehabilitation, sheltered employment or tuberculosis allowance. Although payment is at the same rate as for married people on the age pension, additional payments may be made if the couple have children in their care. Additional payments are normally made to the wife. Supplementary assistance (subject to a separate income test) may be paid if more than $10 a week is paid for rent or lodgings. Spouse carer's pension becomes taxable if a man is 65 or older and a woman 60 or older.

Fringe benefits Pensioners whose other income does not exceed $57 a week if single, or $94 a week combined if married, are entitled to a number of concessions and benefits. These include: Pensioner health benefit card which entitles the holder to free standard ward care in a public hospital and free medical care if the doctor bulk bills; otherwise 85 per cent of the scheduled fee may be reimbursed from Commonwealth Medical Benefits by registering with a private fund; it costs nothing to register. Free eye tests and a reduced rate for spectacles. Free hearing aids and maintenance of the aids. Special concessional rates on ambulance subscription, car registration, telephone rental and public transport. Substantial reduction in local council and Board of Works rates. Concessions at cinemas and theatres and hairdressers are available in many cases.

Domiciliary nursing care benefit This is payable to any person caring for a 'patient' in his or her own home who is also receiving regular nursing care. The current rate of $21 a week is paid towards the costs of home care by the Commonwealth Department of Health. Applications have to be confirmed by a doctor.

Funeral benefits allowance This is paid in respect of a pensioner who was entitled to fringe benefits at the time of death at the rate of $20. If the applicant for the allowance is also a pensioner on fringe benefits, the amount awarded is $40 on provision of a copy of the funeral account.

Special benefits Those caring for sick relatives may be eligible if they satisfy an income test and have no other adequate source of income. This is a discretionary payment to cover circumstances not catered for by other pensions and benefits. To qualify, medical evidence stating that the sick relative requires constant care and attention, because their condition makes them unfit for work, must be provided. Payments are $73.60 as long as other income does not exceed $20.

Meals on wheels Although rates for local councils vary, meals-on-wheels services average $2 a day. A doctor's certificate may be needed.

Home help service A subsidy for visits by a domestic help is available if supported by a medical certificate.

Other community resources Include:

1. Visits by the Royal District Nursing Service, when nurses call regularly to bathe elderly patients, administer injections and dress wounds at the request of a doctor or other health professional; costs are assessed on circumstances.

2. Day hospitals which patients may attend on a regular basis for therapy and to meet other people.

3. Drop-in centres, where, under the sponsorship of local churches, groups are organised for people to socialise.

4. Temporary relief beds. It is sometimes possible to arrange for the temporary care of an elderly person while his carer takes a holiday. Family relief beds are available in major geriatric hospitals but because most are zoned they will take only patients living within their area.

Addendum

We would like to be able to say that in the time since this book was first printed, a cure has been discovered for Alzheimer's Disease. But no medical team has yet been able to perform this miracle.

However, with more government eyes opened to the horrifying dimensions of the affliction there is now greater world-wide concern as to what can be done about the problems of ageing, particularly the dementing aged.

One tremendous step forward came early in 1986 when a team of British doctors announced they had evidence suggesting that aluminium getting into the brain was causing the deterioration. The aluminium theory, of course, is not new. But the medical team believe they have pinpointed how it gets there.

Dr James Edwardson and his colleagues at Newcastle General Hospital in New South Wales looked closely at the aluminium connection after studying reports that some patients undergoing lengthy dialysis treatment developed symptoms similar to Alzheimer's Disease. Aluminium in the tap water used to clean dialysis machines had been examined as a possible culprit and post mortems revealed aluminium in the brains of those who had shown Alzheimer symptoms.

Dr Edwardson and his team, with the aid of space-age nuclear magnetic equipment, were able to pinpoint where aluminium built up in the brain — right in the heart of the deteriorating pieces of nerve cells known as plaques. Convinced that aluminium is the cause rather that the effect of the deterioration, researchers are now continuing to look into the source of the metal traces.

Aluminium is similar to the chemical composition of calcium, of which many older people are found to be deficient. Dr Edwardson suggests that the metabolism of an elderly person tries to balance the deficiency by absorbing more calcium, but in fact in some haywire fashion aluminium is ingested. Already the Newcastle medical team has found that some 30 per cent of elderly people brought to hospital with fractured or broken femurs and calcium deficiency are displaying the symptoms of dementia.

Bibliography

Blakemore, Colin *Mechanics of the Mind* Cambridge University Press, Cambridge, UK, 1977

Clemente, Carmine D. and Lindsley, Donald B., eds *Brain Function*, vol V, *Aggression and Defence* University of California Press, Los Angeles, 1967

Elliott, H. Chandler *The Shape of Intelligence*, Charles Scribner's Sons, New York, 1969

Georgakas, Dan *The Methuselah Factors* Simon & Schuster, New York, 1980

Inglis, Brian *The Diseases of Civilisation* Granada, St Albans, Herts, 1983

Kapust, Lissa Robins *Living with Dementia: The Ongoing Funeral* paper, from Social Work in Health Care, vol 7 (4), 1982 The Haworth Press, Boston, Mass.

Lockhart, R.D., Hamilton, G.F. and Fyfe, F.W. *Anatomy of the Human Body* Faber & Faber, London, 1969

Lynch, Dr James J. *The Broken Heart: The Medical Consequences of Loneliness* Harper & Row, Basic Books, New York, 1977

Mace, Nancy L. and Rabins, Peter V. *The 36-Hour Day* Johns Hopkins University Press, Baltimore, Md. 1981

Moss, Brian *Dementia: Who Cares?* Final Report to the Winston Churchill Memorial Trust, Melbourne, 1984

Noback, Charles R. and Demarest, Robert J. *The Human Nervous System* McGraw-Hill, New York, 1975

Powell, Lenore S. and Courtice, Katie *Alzheimer's Disease: A Guide for Families* Addison-Wesley, Reading, Mass., 1983

Prochazka, Z., Henschke, P., Skinner, E. and Last, P. *Memory Loss and Confusion: Dementia* South Australian Health Commission, Adelaide, 1983

Stevens, Leonard *Explorers of the Brain* Alfred A. Knopf, New York, 1971

Walshe, Sir Francis *Diseases of the Nervous System* Churchill Livingstone, Edinburgh and London, 1973

American Journal of Psychiatry; *British Medical Journal*; *Clinical Gerontologist*, USA; *Community Care*, UK; *Dimensions in Health Service*, Ontario, Canada; *Generations*, Journal of the Western Gerontological Society, California, USA; *Geriatric Medicine*, UK; *Health and Social Services Journal*, UK; *The Health Services*, UK; *International Journal of Nursing Studies*, UK; *Journal of Community Nursing*, UK; *Journal of Family Practice*, USA; *Journal of Medical Ethics*, UK; *Medical Education (International)*, UK; *Medical News Group*, sponsored by Dorsey Laboratories, UK; *Nursing Mirror*, UK; *Nursing Times*, UK; *The Practitioner*, UK; *Research Resources Reporter*, US Department of Health and Human Services; *World Health*, USA

Der Spiegel magazine, Germany; *The Age*, Melbourne; *The Australian*, Sydney; *The Australian Women's Weekly*, Sydney; *The National Times*, Sydney; *New Idea* magazine, Melbourne; *The Sun*, Melbourne; *The Sun-Herald*, Sydney; *The Daily Mail*, London, *The Guardian*, London; *Jewish Chronical*, UK; *The Sunday Times*, London; *Woman* magazine, UK; *The Boston Globe*; *The Chicago Tribune*; *Chicago Sunday Sun Times*; *50 Plus* magazine, USA; *Ladies Home Journal*, USA; *The New York Times*; *Time* magazine, New York; *US News and World Report*; *The Washington Post*